OXFORD PAIN MANAGEMENT LIBRARY

Cancer-related Breakthrough Pain

Second Edition

▶ Except where otherwise stated, drug doses and recommendations are for the non-pregnant adult who is not breast-feeding.

O P M L

OXFORD PAIN MANAGEMENT LIBRARY

Cancer-related Breakthrough Pain

Second Edition

Dr Andrew Davies

Consultant in Palliative Medicine
St. Luke's Cancer Centre
Royal Surrey County Hospital
Guildford
United Kingdom

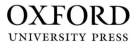

OXFORD
UNIVERSITY PRESS

OXFORD
UNIVERSITY PRESS

Great Clarendon Street, Oxford, OX2 6DP,
United Kingdom

Oxford University Press is a department of the University of Oxford.
It furthers the University's objective of excellence in research, scholarship,
and education by publishing worldwide. Oxford is a registered trade mark of
Oxford University Press in the UK and in certain other countries

First Edition published 2008
Second Edition published 2012

Impression: 1

British Library Cataloguing in Publication Data

Data available

Library of Congress Cataloging in Publication Data

Data available

ISBN 978-0-19-965697-4

Printed in Great Britain by
Ashford Colour Press Ltd., Gosport, Hampshire

25033875

Contents

Preface

The second edition of *Cancer-related breakthrough pain* has been completely re-written to reflect the changes in clinical practice that have occurred over the last 5 years. The format remains much the same, and I would like to thank the original contributors for providing the foundations for the updated version: Fiona Bailey, Nicholas Christelis, Ola Dale, Ann Farley, Jackie Filshie, Craig Gannon, Diane Laverty, Charles Skinner, Emma Thompson, and John Zeppetella.

Dr Andrew Davies
Consultant in Palliative Medicine
Royal Surrey County Hospital NHS Foundation Trust
Guildford
United Kingdom

Symbols and abbreviations

APM	Association for Palliative Medicine of Great Britain and Ireland
BPQ	Breakthrough Pain Questionnaire
BTP	breakthrough pain
FBT	fentanyl buccal tablet
FBSF	fentanyl buccal soluble film
FPNS	fentanyl pectin nasal spray
IASP	International Association for the Study of Pain
IM	intramuscular
INFS	intranasal fentanyl spray
MSIR	morphine sulphate immediate release
NNT	number needed to treat
NSAID	non-steroidal anti-inflammatory drug
ODT	orally disintegrating tablet
OTFC	oral transmucosal fentanyl citrate
PCA	patient controlled analgesia
SC	subcutaneous
TENS	transcutaneous electrical nerve stimulation

Chapter 1

Introduction

'You can't find it [inner peace] in that darkness of pain... I can't emphasize that the pain blinds you to all of that, blinds you to all that's positive. I mean the real bad pain... it just closes you down. You just can't get through it... it's an iron door and it's one thing you don't wanna go through... you just wanna, wanna stop'

(Coyle, 2004)

Key points

- Breakthrough pain is a transient exacerbation of pain that occurs despite relatively stable and adequately controlled background pain
- In the last 20 years there has been an increasing interest in the phenomenon of breakthrough pain
- There is an increasing range of pharmacological options for the treatment of breakthrough pain
- The focus of this book is on cancer-related break-through pain
- Breakthrough pain may also occur in patients with non-malignant diseases.

1.1 Introduction

Over the last 20 years, there has been an increasing interest in the phenomenon of breakthrough pain. This upsurge in interest has been generated by a greater awareness of the problem of break-through pain (secondary to improvements in the management of background pain), and has been fuelled by an increasing range of pharmacological options for the treatment of breakthrough pain (Colleau, 1999).

The focus of this book is on cancer-related breakthrough pain in adults. However, breakthrough pain is also reported to be common in children with cancer (Friedrichsdorf *et al*, 2007), and in adults (and presumably children) with non-malignant diseases associated with acute/chronic pain (Zeppetella *et al*, 2001; Portenoy *et al*, 2006).

1.2 **Definitions**

1.2.1 **Pain**

The standard definition of pain is 'an unpleasant sensory and emotional experience associated with actual or potential tissue damage, or described in terms of such damage' (Merskey and Bogduk, 1994).

1.2.2 **Background pain**

Background pain refers to 'constant or continuous pain of long duration' (Ferrell *et al*, 1999). It should be noted that the phrase 'long duration' refers to a period of $\geq$ 12 hr/day (Ferrell *et al*, 1999).

The term background pain is widely used in the United Kingdom. However, other terms are used in clinical practice and the medical literature to describe the same phenomenon, including 'basal pain', 'baseline pain' and 'persistent pain' (Ferrell et al, 1999).

1.2.3 **Breakthrough pain**

There is no standard definition of breakthrough pain. A recent definition of breakthrough pain is 'a transient exacerbation of pain that occurs either spontaneously, or in relation to a specific predictable or unpredictable trigger, despite relatively stable and adequately controlled background pain' (Davies *et al*, 2009).

The term breakthrough pain is widely used throughout the world. However, other terms are also used in clinical practice and the medical literature to describe the same phenomenon, including 'episodic pain', 'exacerbation of pain', 'pain flare', 'transient pain', and 'transitory pain' (Colleau, 1999).

1.3 **Classification**

Breakthrough pain is usually classified according to its relationship to specific events (Davies *et al*, 2009):

- Spontaneous pain (also known as 'idiopathic pain') – this type of pain occurs unexpectedly
- Incident pain (also known as 'precipitated pain' or, when appropriate, 'movement-related pain') – this type of pain is related to specific events, and can be sub-classified into three categories:
  1. Volitional incident pain – is precipitated by a voluntary act (e.g. walking)

2. Non-volitional incident pain – is precipitated by an involuntary act (e.g. coughing)
3. Procedural pain – is related to a therapeutic intervention (e.g. wound dressing).

In the past, 'end-of-dose failure' was often considered to be a sub-type of breakthrough pain. (End-of-dose failure describes an exacerbation of pain that occurs prior to the next dose of the background analgesic, and reflects declining levels of the background analgesic). However, now many experts believe that end-of-dose failure is not a subtype of breakthrough pain, since they perceive that end-of-dose failure represents 'inadequately' controlled background pain (Davies et al, 2009). Table 1.2 shows the prevalence of breakthrough pain subtypes in English-language studies applying standard criteria for breakthrough pain (Portenoy & Hagen, 1990; Fine & Busch, 1998; Portenoy et al, 1999; Zeppetella et al, 2000; Gomez-Batiste et al, 2002; Hwang et al, 2003; Davies et al, 2011).

1.4 **Epidemiology**

Pain is a common problem in patients with cancer. Indeed, the prevalence of pain has been reported to be 30–40% amongst patients with early disease (receiving anti-cancer therapy), and 70–90% amongst patients with advanced disease (Foley, 2004).

Similarly, breakthrough pain is a common problem in patients with cancer. The prevalence of breakthrough pain has been reported to be 19–95% amongst various groups of patients (Zeppetella & Ribeiro, 2003). This disparity reflects a number of factors, including differences in the definition utilized, in the methods utilized, and in the populations studied (Mercadante et al, 2002). Furthermore, the reporting of breakthrough pain is affected by certain language/geographical variables (see below).

Many authors have adopted the diagnostic criteria for breakthrough pain employed by Portenoy & Hagen (1990). These criteria are: 1) the presence of stable analgesia in the previous 48 hr; 2) the presence of controlled background pain in the previous 24 hr (i.e. average pain intensity of none, mild or moderate for over half of the previous 24 hr); and 3) the presence of 'temporary flares of severe or excruciating pain' in the previous 24 hr.

Table 1.1 shows the prevalence of breakthrough pain in English-language studies applying standard criteria for breakthrough pain (Portenoy & Hagen, 1990; Fine & Busch, 1998; Portenoy et al, 1999; Zeppetella et al, 2000; Fortner et al, 2002; Gomez-Batiste et al, 2002; Fortner et al, 2003; Hwang et al, 2003; Portenoy et al, 2010a). It should be noted that these figures represent the prevalence of breakthrough pain in selected populations of cancer patients, rather

Table 1.1 Prevalence of breakthrough pain in studies applying standard criteria for breakthrough pain

Study	Type of population	Prevalence of breakthrough pain (see comments)	Comments
Portenoy & Hagen, 1990	Hospital inpatients (pain team referrals) – USA n = 90	63%	Criteria for BTP outlined in this study. 90 patients assessed; 63 patients reported controlled background pain; 41 patients reported BTP.
Fine & Busch, 1998	Hospice homecare patients – USA n = 22	86%	Only patients with pain eligible. 22 patients reported background pain; 19 patients reported BTP.
Portenoy et al,1999	Hospital inpatients – USA n = 178	51%	Only patients on regular opioid analgesics eligible. 178 patients assessed; 164 patients reported controlled background pain; 84 patients reported BTP.
Zeppetella et al, 2000	Hospice inpatients – UK n = 414	89%	381 patients assessed (33 patients not assessable); 245 patients reported background pain; 218 patients reported BTP.
Fortner et al, 2002	Cancer patients (home setting) – USA n = 1000	63%	Telephone survey of cancer patients. 1000 patients assessed; 256 patients reported regular analgesic usage; 160 patients reported BTP.

Gomez-Batiste et al, 2002	Palliative care patients (various settings) – Spain n = 407	41%	397 patients assessed (10 patients not assessable); 163 patients reported BTP.
Fortner et al, 2003	Outpatients – USA n = 373	23%	Non-specific data relating to the patients' pain scores/pain medications were used to diagnose presence of BTP. 373 patients assessed; 144 patients reported background pain; 33 patients were deemed to have BTP.
Hwang et al, 2003	VA hospital in/outpatients – USA n = 74	70%	Only patients with pain eligible. 74 patients reported background pain; 52 patients reported BTP. [After a week of treatment, BTP prevalence decreased from 70% to 36%].
Portenoy et al, 2010a	Outpatients – USA n = 78	33%	Only patients on regular opioid analgesics, and with controlled background pain eligible. 78 patients assessed; 26 patients reported BTP

BTP = breakthrough pain; VA = Veterans Affairs.

Table 1.2 Prevalence of breakthrough pain subtypes in studies using standard criteria for breakthrough pain

Study	Breakthrough pain subtypes			Comments
	Spontaneous pain	Incident pain	'End of dose failure'*	
Portenoy & Hagen, 1990	27%	43%	18%	12% pains were 'mixed' in nature (incident and end of dose failure). Incident pain precipitants: movement 22%; coughing 12%; sitting 4%; touch 2%.
Fine & Busch, 1998	No data	~ 50%	No data	No further details in paper.
Portenoy et al, 1999	38%	49%	13%	Incident pain precipitants: movement 27.8%; defaecation 5.7%; urination 3.8%; coughing 3.7%; sitting 3.7%; breathing 1.9%; eating / drinking 1.9%.
Zeppetella et al, 2000	59%	24%	17%	No further details in paper.
Gomez-Batiste et al, 2002	32%	52%	15%	Incident pain precipitants: movement 38%; eating / drinking 3%; defaecation 2%; coughing 2%.
Hwang et al, 2003	17%	64%	19%	Data based on initial assessment of patient. Incident pain precipitants: movement 44%; coughing 4%; eating /drinking 4%; defaecation 2%; sitting 2%.
Davies et al, 2011	39%	44%	n/a	17% pains were 'mixed' in nature (spontaneous and incident). Patients with end of dose failure excluded from study

*'End of dose failure' is now generally not considered to be a subtype of breakthrough pain (Davies et al, 2009).

than the prevalence of breakthrough pain in the general population of cancer patients.

Interestingly, the International Association for the Study of Pain (IASP) survey of cancer pain characteristics and syndromes found that pain specialists from English-speaking (North America, Australasia) and Northern/Western European countries reported more breakthrough pain than pain specialists from South American, Asian and Southern/Eastern European countries (Caraceni & Portenoy, 1999; Caraceni et al, 2004).

Breakthrough pain appears to be more common in patients with advanced disease (Colleau, 2004), in patients with poor performance status (Caraceni et al, 2004), in patients with pain originating from the vertebral column (and to a lesser extent other weight-bearing bones/joints) (Caraceni et al, 2004), and in patients with pain originating from the nerve plexuses (and to a lesser extent nerve roots) (Caraceni et al, 2004).

1.5 **Aetiology**

The aetiology of the breakthrough pain is often the same as that of the background pain (Portenoy & Hagen, 1990; Portenoy et al, 1999). Thus, breakthrough pain may be due to (Zeppetella & Ribeiro, 2003):

- Direct effect of the cancer
- Indirect effect of the cancer (i.e. secondary to disability)
- Effect of the anti-cancer treatment
- Effect of a concomitant illness.

Indeed, breakthrough pain may be experienced by patients with all stages of cancer (at diagnosis, during active treatment, during remission, during relapse/progression, following cure) (Portenoy & Hagen, 1990; Portenoy et al, 1999). Table 1.3 shows the aetiology of breakthrough pain in relevant published studies (Portenoy & Hagen, 1990; Portenoy et al, 1999; Zeppetella et al, 2000).

Not surprisingly, the pathophysiology of the breakthrough pain is also often the same as that of the background pain. Thus, breakthrough pain may be:

- Nociceptive pain – this type of pain is related to stimulation of the nerve endings, and can be sub-classified into two categories:
  1. Somatic pain – originates from the cutaneous/musculoskeletal tissues of the body
  2. Visceral pain – originates from the organs of the body
- Neuropathic pain – this type of pain is related to damage to/dysfunction of the nerve structure
- Mixed pain – a combination of nociceptive and neuropathic pain.

Table 1.3 Aetiology and pathophysiology of breakthrough pain						
Study	Aetiology			Pathophysiology		
	Cancer	Cancer treatment	Concomitant disease	Nociceptive	Neuropathic pain	Mixed pain
Portenoy & Hagen, 1990	76%	20%	4%	53%	27%	20%
Portenoy et al, 1999	65%	35%	0%	38%	10%	52%
Zeppetella et al, 2000	71%	11%	18%	75%	9%	16%

Table 1.3 shows the pathophysiology of breakthrough pain in relevant published studies (Portenoy & Hagen, 1990; Portenoy et al, 1999; Zeppetella et al, 2000).

1.6 Clinical features

Breakthrough pain is not a single entity, but a spectrum of very different entities. The clinical features vary from individual to individual, and may vary within an individual over time (Portenoy, 1997). Nevertheless, breakthrough pain is often reported to be frequent in occurrence, acute in onset, short in duration, and moderate-to-severe in intensity. Moreover, the clinical features of the breakthrough pain are often related to the clinical features of the background pain (Portenoy et al, 1999).

Breakthrough pain may result in a number of other physical, psychological and social problems. Indeed, the presence of breakthrough pain can have a significant negative impact on the activities of daily living (Portenoy et al, 1999; Hwang et al, 2003; Portenoy et al, 2010b; Davies et al, 2011). The degree of interference seems to be related to the characteristics of the breakthrough pain: patients with spontaneous pain (Portenoy et al, 1999), and patients with severe pain (Swanwick et al, 2001), may experience particular problems.

Not surprisingly, breakthrough pain is associated with increased use of healthcare services (i.e. increased outpatient visits, increased inpatient admissions) (Fortner et al, 2002). The result of the increased use of healthcare services is an increase in direct costs (e.g. prescription costs), and in indirect costs (e.g. transportation costs) for both the health service and the patient and their carers (Fortner et al, 2003).

The clinical features of breakthrough pain are discussed in more detail in Chapter 2.

1.7 Conclusion

The quotation at the start of the chapter exemplifies the negative effects of poorly controlled cancer pain (Coyle, 2004), whilst the subsequent quotation (from the same patient) reinforces the positive effects of well controlled cancer pain (Coyle, 2004). Breakthrough pain is a major challenge to healthcare professionals (as well as to their patients). Nevertheless, in some cases, it is possible to eradicate the breakthrough pain (Hwang et al, 2003). Moreover, in all cases, it is should be possible to ameliorate the breakthrough pain. The following chapters will address the issues of the assessment, the general principles of management, and the specific options for management of cancer-related breakthrough pain.

*'Once the pain was relieved it was the most beautiful experience
of my life, to be able to participate and control the pain'*
(Coyle, 2004)

References

Caraceni, A., Portenoy, R.K. (1999) An international survey of cancer pain characteristics and syndromes. *Pain*, **82**, 263–74.

Caraceni, A., Martini, C., Zecca, E. *et al* (2004) Breakthrough pain characteristics and syndromes in patients with cancer pain. An international survey. *Palliative Medicine*, **18**, 177–83.

Colleau, S.M. (1999) The significance of breakthrough pain in cancer. *Cancer Pain Release*, **12**, 1–4.

Colleau, S.M. (2004) Breakthrough (episodic) vs. baseline (persistent) pain in cancer. *Cancer Pain Release*, **17**, 1–3.

Coyle, N. (2004) In their own words: seven advanced cancer patients describe their experience with pain and the use of opioid drugs. *Journal of Pain and Symptom Management*, **27**, 300–9.

Davies, A.N., Dickman, A., Reid, C., Stevens, A.M., Zeppetella, G. (2009) The management of cancer-related breakthrough pain: recommendations of a task group of the Science Committee of the Association for Palliative Medicine of Great Britain and Ireland. *European Journal of Pain*, **13**, 331–8.

Davies, A., Zeppetella, G., Andersen, S. *et al* (2011). Multi-centre European study of breakthrough cancer pain: pain characteristics and patient perceptions of current and potential management strategies. *European Journal of Pain*, **15**, 756–63.

Ferrell, B.R., Juarez, G., Borneman, T. (1999) Use of routine and breakthrough analgesia in home care. *Oncology Nursing Forum*, **26**, 1655–61.

Fine, P.G., Busch, M.A. (1998). Characterization of breakthrough pain by hospice patients and their caregivers. *Journal of Pain and Symptom Management*, **16**, 179–83.

Foley, K.M. (2004) Acute and chronic cancer pain syndromes. In Doyle, D., Hanks, G., Cherny, N., Calman, K., ed. *Oxford Textbook of Palliative Medicine*, 3rd edn, pp. 298–316. Oxford University Press, Oxford.

Fortner, B.V., Okon, T.A., Portenoy, R.K. (2002) A survey of pain-related hospitalizations, emergency department visits, and physician office visits reported by cancer patients with and without history of breakthrough pain. *Journal of Pain*, **3**, 38–44.

Fortner, B.V., Demarco, G., Irving, G. *et al* (2003) Description and predictors of direct and indirect costs of pain reported by cancer patients. *Journal of Pain and Symptom Management*, **25**, 9–18.

Friedrichsdorf, S.J., Finney, D., Bergin, M., Stevens, M., Collins, J.J. (2007) Breakthrough pain in children with cancer. *Journal of Pain and Symptom Management*, **34**, 209–16.

Gómez-Batiste, X., Madrid, F., Moreno, F. *et al* (2002). Breakthrough cancer pain: prevalence and characteristics in patients in Catalonia, Spain. *Journal of Pain and Symptom Management*, **24**, 45–52.

Hwang, S.S., Chang, V.T., Kasimis, B. (2003) Cancer breakthrough pain characteristics and responses to treatment at a VA medical center. *Pain*, **101**, 55–64.

Mercadante, S., Radbruch, L., Caraceni, A. *et al* (2002) Episodic (breakthrough) pain. Consensus conference of an Expert Working Group of the European Association for Palliative Care. *Cancer*, **94**, 832–9.

Merskey, H., Bogduk, N. (1994) *Classification of Chronic Pain*, 2nd edn. IASP Press, Seattle, 209–14.

Portenoy, R.K., Hagen, N.A. (1990) Breakthrough pain: definition, prevalence and characteristics. *Pain*, **41**, 273–81.

Portenoy, R.K. (1997) Treatment of temporal variations in chronic cancer pain. *Seminars in Oncology*, **5**, S16–7-12.

Portenoy, R.K., Payne, D., Jacobsen, P. (1999) Breakthrough pain: characteristics and impact in patients with cancer pain. *Pain*, **81**, 129–34.

Portenoy, R.K., Bennett, D.S., Rauck, R. *et al* (2006) Prevalence and characteristics of breakthrough pain in opioid-treated patients with chronic noncancer pain. *Journal of Pain*, **7**, 583–91.

Portenoy, R.K., Bruns, D., Shoemaker, B., Shoemaker, S.A. (2010a) Breakthrough pain in community-dwelling patients with cancer pain and noncancer pain, Part 1: prevalence and characteristics. *Journal of Opioid Management*, **6**, 97–108.

Portenoy, R.K., Bruns, D., Shoemaker, B., Shoemaker, S.A. (2010b) Breakthrough pain in community-dwelling patients with cancer pain and noncancer pain, Part 2: impact on function, mood, and quality of life. *Journal of Opioid Management*, **6**, 109–16.

Swanwick, M., Haworth, M., Lennard, R.F. (2001) The prevalence of episodic pain in cancer: a survey of hospice patients on admission. *Palliative Medicine*, **15**, 9–18.

Zeppetella, G., O'Doherty, C.A., Collins, S. (2000) Prevalence and characteristics of breakthrough pain in cancer patients admitted to a hospice. *Journal of Pain and Symptom Management*, **20**, 87–92.

Zeppetella, G., O'Doherty, C.A., Collins, S. (2001) Prevalence and characteristics of breakthrough pain in patients with non-malignant terminal disease admitted to a hospice. *Palliative Medicine*, **15**, 243–6.

Zeppetella, G., Ribeiro, M.D. (2003) Pharmacotherapy of cancer-related episodic pain. *Expert Opinion on Pharmacotherapy*, **4**, 493–502.

Chapter 2

Clinical features

Key points

- Breakthrough pain is very diverse in nature
- Breakthrough pain can have multiple causes with multiple pathophysiologies
- Breakthrough pain can present with numerous clinical features and numerous complications
- Breakthrough pain is a cause of significant morbidity in many cases
- The ability to cope with breakthrough pain seems to be related to the underlying aetiology
- Patients with cancer-related pain may have more problems coping than patients with cancer treatment-related pain.

2.1 Introduction

Breakthrough pain has been defined as 'a transient exacerbation of pain that occurs either spontaneously, or in relation to a specific predictable or unpredictable trigger, despite relatively stable and adequately controlled background pain' (Davies et al, 2009). This definition is very broad, and reflects the fact that breakthrough pain is very diverse in nature. Thus, breakthrough pain can have multiple causes with multiple pathophysiologies, and can present with numerous clinical features and numerous complications. In some cases, breakthrough pain is a mere inconvenience, but in many cases breakthrough pain is a cause of significant morbidity.

2.2 Classification

As discussed in Chapter 1, breakthrough pain can be classified according to its relationship to specific events (Davies et al, 2009):

- Spontaneous pain (also known as 'idiopathic pain') – this type of pain occurs unexpectedly

- Incident pain (also known as 'precipitated pain' or, when appropriate, 'movement-related pain') – this type of pain is related to specific events, and can be sub-classified into three categories:
  1. Volitional incident pain – is precipitated by a voluntary act (e.g. walking)
  2. Non-volitional incident pain – is precipitated by an involuntary act (e.g. coughing)
  3. Procedural pain – is related to a therapeutic intervention (e.g. wound dressing).

Table 1.2 shows the breakdown of the different types of breakthrough pain in English language studies that have applied standard criteria for diagnosing breakthrough pain (Portenoy & Hagen, 1990; Fine & Busch, 1998; Portenoy *et al*, 1999; Zeppetella *et al*, 2000; Gómez-Batiste *et al*, 2002; Hwang *et al*, 2003; Davies *et al*, 2011). Boxes 2.1 and 2.2 (supported by Figures 2.1 and 2.2) illustrate case histories from patients with the different types of breakthrough pain.

> **Box 2.1 Case history of patient with spontaneous type breakthrough pain**
>
> Mr PW is a 50 year old gentleman with localized Ewing's sarcoma of the sacrum (Figure 2.1). He presented to the palliative care team with severe pain in the penis/scrotum secondary to the primary tumour. This pain was intermittent in nature, occurring 3–4 times per hour, and lasting < 1 min per episode. (There were no precipitating/aggravating factors.) He also complained of moderate pain in the gluteal area/legs secondary to the primary tumour. This pain was persistent in nature. The patient had been receiving paracetamol and low doses of gabapentin for the pain.
>
> The paracetamol was replaced by co-codamol 30/500, which resulted in good control of the persistent pain. (The co-codamol 30/500 had no effect on the spontaneous pain.) In addition, the gabapentin was titrated upwards, which resulted in good control of the spontaneous pain. During this period, the patient also received an epidural injection of steroid (which had little effect on the pain), and a course of radical radiotherapy to the sacrum (which initially aggravated the pain). In due course, following completion of multimodal oncological therapy, the patient was able to discontinue all of the aforementioned analgesics.

2.3 **General features**

Breakthrough pain is not a single entity, but a spectrum of very different entities. The clinical features vary from individual to individual,

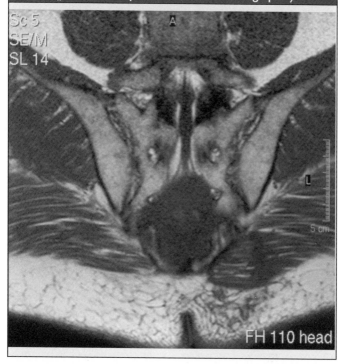

Fig 2.1 MRI scan showing primary Ewing's sarcoma involving sacrum (patient with spontaneous breakthrough pain)

and may vary within an individual over time (Portenoy, 1997; Mercadante et al, 2010). However, the clinical features of the breakthrough pain are often related to the clinical features of the background pain (Portenoy et al, 1999). Tables 2.1 and 2.2 show some of the characteristics of breakthrough pain in English language studies that have applied standard criteria for diagnosing breakthrough pain (Portenoy & Hagen, 1990; Fine & Busch, 1998; Portenoy et al, 1999; Zeppetella et al, 2000; Gómez-Batiste et al, 2002; Hwang et al, 2003; Davies et al, 2011).

The diagnosis of breakthrough pain depends on the presence of well controlled background pain, and so the initial presentation of the breakthrough pain often coincides with the successful management of the background pain. The development/progression of breakthrough pain may signify the progression of underlying pathology, or the development of new pathology (e.g. pathological fracture) (Patt & Ellison, 1998). However, the development/progression of breakthrough pain may also signify problems relating to the analgesic regimen (e.g. development of tolerance) (Patt & Ellison, 1998).

Box 2.2 Case history of patient with incident type breakthrough pain

Mr ML was a 64 year old gentleman with advanced renal cell carcinoma. He had widespread bone metastases, including disease in the thoracic spine, lumbar spine and the pelvis (particularly the left acetabulum: Figure 2.2). He complained of low back and hip pains, which were present at rest, but were more severe on movement. As a result of the incident pain, he was rendered bed bound. Moreover, movement in the bed also resulted in significant pain.

He was started on normal-release morphine sulphate, and the dose was gradually titrated upwards in an attempt to control the pain. The pain at rest was well controlled, but the pain on movement remained uncontrolled, and further titration of the morphine resulted in the development of opioid toxicity. The morphine was switched to oxycodone, but although the opioid toxicity settled, the pain on movement remained uncontrolled.

An epidural catheter was inserted, and an infusion of fentanyl and bupivacaine commenced. This resulted in excellent pain relief, so much so that the patient was able to get out of bed and sit in a chair. Subsequently, following a course of palliative radiotherapy to the lumbar spine, the epidural was able to be removed, and conventional analgesics reinstated (paracetamol, oxycodone).

Fig 2.2 X-ray showing metastatic renal cell carcinoma involving acetabulum (patient with incident breakthrough pain)

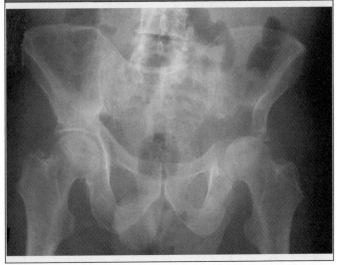

Table 2.1 Characteristics of breakthrough pain in studies applying standard criteria for breakthrough pain

Study	BTP* connected to background pain	Number types BTP	Number episodes BTP (episodes/day)	Comments
Portenoy & Hagen, 1990	96%	1 pain – 78% 2 pains – 20% 3 pains – 2%	Median – 4 (range 1–3600)	The patient with 3600 episodes/day had a rib fracture and a persistent cough.
Fine & Busch, 1998	–	–	Mean 2.9 (range 1–5.5)	
Portenoy et al, 1999	100%	1 pain – 83.1% 2 pains – 14.5% 3 pains – 2.4%	Median 6 (range 1–60)	
Zeppetella et al, 2000	89%	Mean 2 pains (range 1–5)	Mean 4 (range 1–14)	
Gómez-Batiste et al, 2002	–	–	Mean 1.5 (range 0–5)	
Hwang et al, 2003	75%	1 pain – 79% ≥2 pains – 21%	Median 5 (range 1–50)	Data based on initial assessment of patients.
Portenoy et al, 2010	–	1 pain – 100%	Median 1 (range 0–4)	
Davies et al, 2011	–	–	Median 3 (range 0–24)	

BTP – breakthrough pain

Table 2.2 Characteristics of breakthrough pain in studies applying standard criteria for breakthrough pain

Study	Duration BTP (min)	Characteristics BTP (temporal)	Characteristics BTP (intensity)	Comments
Portenoy & Hagen, 1990	Median duration – 30 (range 1–240)	Rapid onset – 43% Gradual onset – 57%	Severe/excruciating – 100%	Only patients with severe or excruciating pain classified as having BTP.
Fine & Busch, 1998	Mean duration – 52 (range <1–240)	-	Mean intensity – 7/10 (range 3/10–10/10)	
Portenoy et al, 1999	-	Median time to peak intensity – 3 min (range <1–30 min)	Severe/ excruciating – 100%	Only patients with severe or excruciating pain classified as having BTP.
Zeppetella et al, 2000	73% episodes – ≤ 30	Rapid onset – 49% Gradual onset – 51%	Slight –16% Moderate – 46% Severe – 36% Excruciating – 2%	

Gómez-Batiste et al, 2002	Mean duration – 33.8 (range 1–180)	Rapid onset – 60% Gradual onset – 39% (Not recorded – 1%)	Median intensity – 8 /10 (range 2/10–10/10)	
Hwang et al, 2003	Median duration – 15 (range 1–120)	Rapid onset – 62% Gradual onset – 38%	Severe/ excruciating – 94%	Only patients with severe or excruciating pain classified as having BTP.
Portenoy et al, 2010a	Median duration – 45 (range 5–360)	Median time to peak intensity – 1 min (range <1–60 min)	Severe – 62% Excruciating – 38%	Only patients with severe or excruciating pain classified as having BTP.
Davies et al, 2011	Median duration – 60 (range <1–480)	Median time to peak intensity – 15 min (range <1–240 min)	Mild – 3% Moderate – 37% Severe – 60%	

Some investigators have reported no relationship between clinical features and the different types of breakthrough pain (i.e. spontaneous pain, incident pain) (Portenoy & Hagen, 1990). However, others have reported that incident pains tend to be rapid in onset (i.e. incident pain – 76%; spontaneous pain – 52%), and tend to have a shorter median duration of action (i.e. incident pain – 20 min; spontaneous pain – 30 min) (Gómez-Batiste et al, 2002). The data on speed of onset has been confirmed in a recent multicentre study; the median time to reach peak intensity for incident pains was 10 min, whilst the median time to reach peak intensity for spontaneous pains was 20 min (Davies et al, 2011).

Similarly, some investigators have reported no relationship between clinical features and the different pathophysiologies of breakthrough pain (i.e. nociceptive, neuropathic) (Portenoy & Hagen, 1990). However, others have reported that neuropathic pains tend to have a shorter duration of action (i.e. neuropathic pain – 91% < 30 min; somatic – 69% < 30 min; visceral – 62% < 30 min) (Zeppetella et al, 2000). It should be noted that patients with different pain pathophysiologies tend to report similar pain qualities. Thus, patients with nociceptive pain report 'burning', 'scalding', 'shooting' and 'pricking' pains as much as patients with neuropathic pain (Rasmussen et al, 2004).

2.4 **Other features**

2.4.1 **Chronobiology of breakthrough pain**

It appears that there is a circadian variation in the intensity of background pain in patients with cancer (Labrecque & Vanier, 1995). Thus, various studies have demonstrated a reduction in the intensity of background pain during the night/early morning (Wilder-Smith et al, 1992a; Wilder-Smith et al, 1992b).

It appears that there is also a circadian variation in the occurrence of breakthrough pain in patients with cancer. For example, Fine & Busch reported that 86% patients experienced breakthrough pain during the day, whilst only 45% patients experienced breakthrough pain during the night (Fine & Busch, 1998). In addition, various studies have demonstrated a reduction in the usage of breakthrough medication during the night/early morning (Bruera et al, 1992, Citron et al, 1992).

The reasons for the circadian variation in breakthrough pain have yet to be determined. However, patients are generally less active during the night and so less likely to experience incident pain during this time. Furthermore, there appears to be a circadian variation in the metabolism of certain analgesics (e.g. morphine), which may be of significance with regard to the control of pain (Gourlay et al, 1995).

Interestingly, delirium results in an alteration in the circadian variation in breakthrough pain. Thus, Gagnon et al reported that patients without delirium used breakthrough medication more often during the day, whilst patients with delirium used breakthrough medication more often during the evening (Gagnon et al, 2001). It should be noted that patients with delirium are often more active during the evening/night, and so more likely to experience volitional (movement-related) incident pain at these times.

2.4.2 Complications of breakthrough pain

Breakthrough pain can result in a number of physical, psychological and social sequelae:

2.4.2.1 Physical complications

Breakthrough pain may be associated with a variety of physical problems. Patients may have difficulty mobilizing (Hwang et al, 2003; Portenoy et al, 1999; Portenoy et al, 2010; Davies et al, 2011), which may lead them to avoid such movement. As a result, they may develop a range of other physical problems, including joint stiffness, muscle wasting, pressure sores, constipation, venous thromboembolism, and pneumonia. Patients may also have difficulty sleeping (Hwang et al, 2003; Portenoy et al, 1999; Portenoy et al, 2010).

2.4.2.2 Psychological complications

The presence of breakthrough pain has been linked to 'lack of enjoyment of life' (Hwang et al, 2003; Portenoy et al, 1999; Portenoy et al, 2010; Davies et al, 2011), and to the presence of mood disturbance (Hwang et al, 2003; Portenoy et al, 1999; Portenoy et al, 2010; Davies et al, 2011), anxiety (Portenoy et al, 1999) and depression (Portenoy et al, 1999). The aetiology of these problems, include the presence of pain, the 'meaning' of the pain, the physical complications of the pain, and the social complications of the pain. Patients also report problems with interpersonal relationships (Hwang et al, 2003; Portenoy et al, 1999; Portenoy et al, 2010; Davies et al, 2011).

2.4.2.3 Social complications

Breakthrough pain may be associated with a variety of social problems. Patients may be unable to work (Hwang et al, 2003; Portenoy et al, 1999; Davies et al, 2011), which may result in financial hardship (and reduced self-esteem). Moreover, patients may have difficulty undertaking the basic activities of daily living, which may necessitate increased input from their family, health services, and social services (and again reduced self-esteem).

Patients may become somewhat isolated, because of difficulty in mobilizing (and so difficulty in socializing). Social isolation is another recognized risk factor for the development of clinical depression.

It can be seen that the presence of breakthrough pain can have a significant negative impact on quality of life. The degree of interference seems in part to be related to the characteristics of the breakthrough pain: patients with spontaneous pain (Portenoy et al, 1999), and patients with severe pain (Swanwick et al, 2000), may experience particular problems. In addition, the ability to cope with breakthrough pain seems in part to be related to the underlying aetiology of the breakthrough pain: patients with cancer-related pain (with all the associated implications) may have more problems coping than patients with cancer treatment-related pain (Foley, 1985).

References

Bruera, E., Macmillan, K., Kuehn, N., Miller, M.J. (1992) Circadian distribution of extra doses of narcotic analgesics in patients with cancer pain: a preliminary report. *Pain*, **49**, 311–4.

Citron, M.L., Kalra, J.M., Seltzer, V.L., Chen, S., Hoffman, M., Walczak, M.B. (1992) Patient-controlled analgesia for cancer pain: a long term study of inpatient and outpatient use. *Cancer Investigation*, **10**, 335–41.

Davies, A.N., Dickman, A., Reid, C., Stevens, A.M., Zeppetella, G. (2009) The management of cancer-related breakthrough pain: recommendations of a task group of the Science Committee of the Association for Palliative Medicine of Great Britain and Ireland. *European Journal of Pain*, **13**, 331–8.

Davies, A., Zeppetella, G., Andersen, S. et al (2011) Multi-centre study of breakthrough cancer pain: pain characteristics and patient perceptions of current and potential management strategies. *European Journal of Pain*, **15**, 756–63.

Fine, P.G., Busch, M.A. (1998) Characterization of breakthrough pain by hospice patients and their caregivers. *Journal of Pain and Symptom Management*, **16**, 179–83.

Foley, K.M. (1985) The treatment of cancer pain. *New England Journal of Medicine*, **313**, 84–95.

Gagnon, B., Lawlor, P.G., Mancini, I.L., Pereira, J.L., Hanson, J., Bruera, E.D. (2001) The impact of delirium on the circadian distribution of breakthrough analgesia in advanced cancer patients. *Journal of Pain and Symptom Management*, **22**, 826–33.

Gómez-Batiste, X., Madrid, F., Moreno, F. et al (2002) Breakthrough cancer pain: prevalence and characteristics in patients in Catalonia, Spain. *Journal of Pain and Symptom Management*, **24**, 45–52.

Gourlay, G.K., Plummer, J.L., Cherry, D.A. (1995) Chronopharmacokinetic variability in plasma morphine concentrations following oral doses of morphine solution. *Pain*, **61**, 375–81.

Hwang, S.S., Chang, V.T., Kasimis, B. (2003) Cancer breakthrough pain characteristics and responses to treatment at a VA medical center. *Pain*, **101**, 55–64.

Labrecque, G., Vanier, M.C. (1995) Biological rhythms in pain and in the effects of opioid analgesics. *Pharmacology and Therapeutics*, **68**, 129–47.

Mercadante, S., Zagonel, V., Breda, E. *et al* (2010) Breakthrough pain in oncology: a longitudinal study. *Journal of Pain and Symptom Management*, **40**, 183–90.

Patt, R.B., Ellison, N.M. (1998) Breakthrough pain in cancer patients: characteristics, prevalence, and treatment. *Oncology* (Huntington), **12**, 1035–52.

Portenoy, R.K., Hagen, N.A. (1990) Breakthrough pain: definition, prevalence and characteristics. *Pain*, **41**, 273–81.

Portenoy, R.K. (1997) Treatment of temporal variations in chronic cancer pain. *Seminars in Oncology*, **5**, S16–7-12.

Portenoy, R.K., Payne, D., Jacobsen, P. (1999) Breakthrough pain: characteristics and impact in patients with cancer pain. *Pain*, **81**, 129–34.

Portenoy, R.K., Bruns, D., Shoemaker, B., Shoemaker, S.A. (2010a) Breakthrough pain in community-dwelling patients with cancer pain and noncancer pain, Part 1: prevalence and characteristics. *Journal of Opioid Management*, **6**, 97–108.

Portenoy, R.K., Bruns, D., Shoemaker, B., Shoemaker, S.A. (2010b) Breakthrough pain in community-dwelling patients with cancer pain and noncancer pain, Part 2: impact on function, mood, and quality of life. *Journal of Opioid Management*, **6**, 109–16.

Rasmussen, P.V., Sindrup, S.H., Jensen, T.S., Bach, F.W. (2004) Symptoms and signs in patients with suspected neuropathic pain. *Pain*, **110**, 461–9.

Swanwick, M., Haworth, M., Lennard, R.F. (2001) The prevalence of episodic pain in cancer: a survey of hospice patients on admission. *Palliative Medicine*, **15**, 9–18.

Wilder-Smith, C.H., Schimke, J., Bettiga, A. (1992a) Circadian pain responses with tramadol (T), a short-acting opioid and alpha-adrenergic agonist, and morphine (M) in cancer pain; presented at the 5th International Conference on Chronopharmacology, July 1992.

Wilder-Smith, C.H., Wilder-Smith, O.H. (1992b) Diurnal patterns of pain in cancer patients during treatment with long-acting opioid; presented at the 5th International Conference on Chronopharmacology, July 1992.

Zeppetella, G., O'Doherty, C.A., Collins, S. (2000) Prevalence and characteristics of breakthrough pain in cancer patients admitted to a hospice. *Journal of Pain and Symptom Management*, **20**, 87–92.

Chapter 3

Assessment

> **Key points**
> - Successful management of breakthrough pain depends on adequate assessment
> - Following assessment, appropriate treatment and adequate reassessment are also important
> - Inadequate assessment may lead to ineffective or even inappropriate treatment
> - The objectives of assessment are to determine pain aetiology and pathophysiology, and factors that indicate or contraindicate particular treatments
> - Assessment of breakthrough pain is essentially the same as the assessment of background pain
> - Inadequate reassessment may lead to the continuance of ineffective or inappropriate treatment.

3.1 Introduction

The successful management of breakthrough pain depends on adequate assessment, appropriate treatment, and adequate reassessment (i.e. assessment of the treatment) (Davies, 2002). Inadequate assessment may lead to utilization of ineffective treatment, or even inappropriate treatment. Similarly, inadequate reassessment may lead to continuance of ineffective/inappropriate treatment (and continuance of pain).

The objectives of assessment are to determine the aetiology of the pain (e.g. cancer-related, non-cancer-related), the pathophysiology of the pain (i.e. nociceptive, neuropathic, mixed), and factors that would indicate/contraindicate particular treatment strategies (e.g. performance status, co-morbidity). The assessment of breakthrough pain is essentially the same as the assessment of background pain.

3.2 **Diagnosis of breakthrough pain**

Recently, a task group of the Association for Palliative Medicine of Great Britain and Ireland suggested a revised definition for break-through pain (i.e. 'a transient exacerbation of pain that occurs either spontaneously, or in relation to a specific predictable or unpredict-able trigger, despite relatively stable and adequately controlled back-ground pain') (Davies *et al*, 2009).

It is important to differentiate patients with uncontrolled back-ground pain experiencing transient exacerbations of that pain from patients with controlled background pain experiencing episodes of breakthrough pain. Thus, the optimal management of the former scenario is likely to be completely different from the optimal man-agement of the latter scenario. Moreover, adequate management of the uncontrolled background pain in the former scenario may lead to the elimination of the transient exacerbations of pain.

The task group of the Association for Palliative Medicine of Great Britain and Ireland also suggested a revised diagnostic criteria for break-through pain (Figure 3.1) (Davies *et al*, 2009; Davies *et al*, 2010).

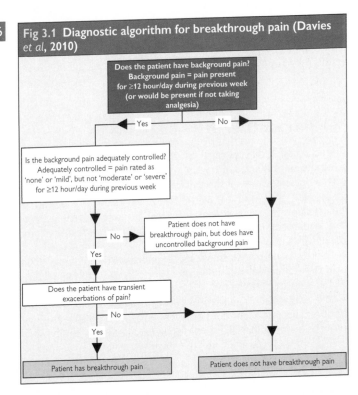

Fig 3.1 **Diagnostic algorithm for breakthrough pain (Davies *et al*, 2010)**

3.3 Assessment of breakthrough pain

The assessment of pain primarily depends on basic clinical skills, i.e. taking a detailed history and performing a thorough examination (Davies, 2002). It is important to take a general history, as well as a pain history. In particular, patients should be screened for psychological, spiritual, and social factors that may be contributing to their experience of pain (the concept of 'total pain') (Twycross, 1994). Similarly, it is important to perform a general examination, as well as an examination of the painful area. Investigations can be extremely useful in the assessment of pain. Nevertheless, investigations should only be viewed as a part of the assessment process, rather than the main focus of the assessment process. Thus, investigations may produce both false negative results, and false positive results.

All patients require a detailed pain history to be taken. The features of the pain that need to be determined include (Foley, 2004):

- Onset of pain
- Temporal pattern of pain — it is important to determine the temporal pattern of the pain, particularly the duration of pain, since this will determine the suitability of certain symptomatic treatments
- Site of pain
- Radiation of pain
- Quality (character) of pain — the quality of the pain may help to determine the aetiology of the pain. However, studies suggest that patients with different pain pathophysiologies tend to report similar pain qualities. Thus, patients with nociceptive pain report 'burning', 'scalding', 'shooting', and pricking' pains as much as patients with neuropathic pain (Rasmussen *et al*, 2004)
- Intensity (severity) of pain
- Exacerbating factors
- Relieving factors
- Response to analgesics — it is essential to determine the response to previous analgesics, and particularly the response to opioid analgesics
- Response to other interventions — it is essential to determine the response to previous anticancer treatment, and to previous non-pharmacological interventions
- Associated physical symptoms — the presence of other symptoms may help to determine the aetiology of the pain. For example, the presence of neurological symptoms suggests an underlying neuropathic component to the pain (e.g. sensory disturbance) (Bennett, 2001)

- Associated psychological symptoms
- Interference with activities of daily living – it is important to ascertain the global impact of the pain. (Activities of daily living can be used as a surrogate marker of the response to treatment).

All patients require a thorough examination to be performed. The examination should include a neurological examination of the relevant area, since the presence of neurological signs suggests an underlying neuropathic component to the pain (Bennett, 2001). It can be useful to reproduce the patient's pain by using so-called 'provocative manoeuvres' (e.g. palpation, passive movement) (Hagen, 1999). However, it is important that the benefits of such manoeuvres (i.e. improved understanding of the pain) outweigh the costs of these manoeuvres (i.e. causation of the pain).

It should be noted that many patients have more than one type of breakthrough pain (Portenoy & Hagen, 1990; Portenoy *et al*, 1999). Each breakthrough pain should be individually assessed, since each breakthrough pain may require a different form of treatment.

3.4 **Reassessment of breakthrough pain**

The primary objective of reassessment is to determine the efficacy and tolerability of any therapeutic intervention. A further objective of reassessment is the identification of significant changes in the breakthrough pain. For example, increasing pain in a bone may represent impending fracture of that bone (which may necessitate a more intensive therapeutic intervention e.g. surgical stabilization).

Various outcome measures have been used to assess the efficacy of therapeutic interventions, including: a) intensity of pain; b) distress of pain; c) pain relief; d) satisfaction with treatment; e) improvement in function; and e) improvement in quality of life (Davies, 2002). The different outcome measures relate to different aspects of the pain. Consequently, there is often a poor correlation between the results obtained with different outcome measures. For example, in one study involving Oncology patients, the percentage of subjects that were 'inadequately treated' varied from 16–91% depending on the specific outcome measure used (de Wit *et al*, 1999).

All of the aforementioned outcome measures have limitations. For example, pain relief is related to the change in pain intensity over a period of time, i.e. it is dependent on the patient's recollection of the baseline pain intensity. There is little consensus on the specific outcome measure that should be used to assess treatment response (de Wit *et al*, 1999). Nevertheless, it is important that a (suitable) outcome measure is used to assess treatment response in all patients (Davies, 2002).

Box 3.1 Examples of pain management scales

Verbal rating scale, e.g. McGill Pain Questionnaire (Melzack, 1975).

No pain; mild; discomforting; distressing; horrible; excruciating

Numerical rating scale, e.g. Brief Pain Inventory (Daut et al, 1983).

A. Pain intensity

0	1	2	3	4	5	6	7	8	9	10

No pain

Pain as bad as you can imagine

B. Pain relief

0% 10% 20% 30% 40% 50% 60% 70% 80% 90% 100%

No relief

Complete relief

Visual analogue scale, e.g. Memorial Pain Assessment Card (Fishman et al, 1987).

A. Pain intensity

LEAST possible pain_____**WORST possible pain**

B. Pain relief

NO relief of pain_____**COMPLETE relief of pain**

Outcome measures are usually based on either a verbal rating scale, a numerical rating scale, or a visual analogue scale (Figure 3.2). Studies have shown a good correlation between the results obtained with these different scales (McQuay & Moore, 1998): the relationship between the results obtained with these different scales is shown in Table 3.1. However, patients with advanced cancer often have difficulty in completing such outcome measures. For example, in one study involving Palliative Care inpatients, 45% of the subjects were unable to complete any of the outcome measures (mainly because of cognitive impairment) (Shannon et al, 1995).

Table 3.1 Correlation between results of different pain measurement scales

Verbal rating scale	Numerical rating scale (0 – 10) (Serlin et al, 1995)	Visual analogue scale (100 mm) (Collins et al, 1997)
None	0	–
Mild	1–4	–
Moderate	5–6	> 30 mm (mean 49)
Severe	7–10	> 54 mm (mean 75)

It should be noted that studies suggest that the formal measurement of pain leads to the improved management of pain. For example, in one study involving Oncology outpatients, subjects whose outcome measures were reviewed were more likely to have had an improvement in their background pain intensity at follow up than subjects whose outcome measures were unavailable for review (Trowbridge et al, 1997).

3.5 Assessment tools

A number of different tools have been developed for the assessment of cancer-related pain (Caraceni et al, 2002). However, these tools invariably focus on the background pain rather than the breakthrough pain. Moreover, most of these tools provide little, or no, information about the breakthrough pain.

Portenoy and Hagen developed the Breakthrough Pain Questionnaire (BPQ) to specifically assess breakthrough pain (Portenoy & Hagen, 1990). The tool enables the healthcare professional to identify patients with breakthrough pain, as well as to collect information about the nature of the breakthrough pain (and of the background pain). The BPQ has not been formally validated, although it has been used in a number of clinical studies (Portenoy & Hagen, 1990; Portenoy et al, 1999). Of note, the BPQ has changed/developed over the years (Russell Portenoy, personal communication).

Hagen and colleagues developed the Alberta Breakthrough Pain Assessment Tool to specifically assess breakthrough pain in the research setting (Hagen et al, 2009). The tool is shown in Figure 3.2. The Alberta Breakthrough Pain Assessment Tool has been validated to a limited degree, and is currently undergoing further investigation/validation. Other examples of breakthrough pain assessment tools are the Episodic (Breakthrough) Pain Documentation Sheet (Zeppetella & Ribeiro, 2002), and the newly developed Breakthrough Pain Assessment Tool (BAT) (Webber et al, 2010).

Fig 3.2 Section of Alberta Breakthrough Pain Assessment Tool

(Reprinted from *Journal of Pain and Symptom Management*, 35:2, Neil A. Hagen, Carla Stiles, Cheryl Nekolaichuk, et al, The Alberta Breakthrough Pain Assessment Tool for Cancer Patients. Copyright (2008), with permission from U.S. Cancer Pain Relief Committee.)

TO BE COMPLETED BY PHYSICIAN OR NURSE

Instructions:

1. This module should be completed with the patient due to its complexity. The patient or clinician can answer the questions in writing, but if completed by the patient, it must be done under close supervision and help must be immediately available if required.

2. The goal is to have the patient characterize up to three distinct types of breakthrough pain. **To do this, define baseline and breakthrough pain for the patient.** Baseline pain can be defined as "the usual, steady pain you always experience." Breakthrough pain can be defined as "a brief flare-up of pain. It can be a flare-up of the usual, steady pain you always experience (your baseline pain) OR it can be a pain that is different from your baseline pain".

3. First ask the patient to describe his or her baseline pain, which may include a description of the location, severity, quality, or other features of this pain, and complete the table below.

4. Then ask how many different types of **breakthrough pains** he/she typically experiences **in a 24 hour period**. A patient may initially distinguish between breakthrough pains on the basis of any of the following variables: location, provocation, quality, etiology, or any other variable the patient feels is important.

5. Ask the patient to identify up to three of his/her **most bothersome breakthrough pains**, and complete the table below; these breakthrough pains will be the ones that are characterized.

6. Please photocopy the subsequent pages of this module to individually characterize each of the patient's three most bothersome breakthrough pains. Note that a separate Module III should be completed for each of the patient's most bothersome breakthrough pains.

Description of baseline pain	
Describe your baseline pain.	

Descriptions of distinct types of breakthrough pain	
What is your most bothersome breakthrough pain?	
What is your second most bothersome breakthrough pain?	
What is your third most bothersome breakthrough pain?	

Q2. Current breakthrough pain medications: list trade name of formulations [list generic names for all opioid and non-opioid analgesics]	Treatment Regimen		
	Route of Administration	Dose	prn Schedule

TO BE COMPLETED BY PATIENT

For which breakthrough pain are you completing this form?	

Q1. Relationship to baseline pain Is this pain a brief flare up of your baseline pain or is it a pain that is different from your baseline pain?	☐ Brief flare up of baseline pain ☐ Different from baseline pain ☐ Not sure
Q2. Last time experienced (a) When did you last have this breakthrough pain? (Please refer to your most recent breakthrough pain experience, regardless of whether or not you took medication for it.)	☐ Today ☐ Yesterday ☐ Before then
(b) Beginning at what time, approximately?	
Q3. Frequency (a) Approximately how many times in the past 24 hours have you had this breakthrough pain? (Please include ALL breakthrough pain experiences, regardless of whether or not you took medication for them.)	
(b) During the past 24 hours is this about the usual for you?	☐ Usual ☐ Better ☐ Worse

31

Q4. Intensity of pain at peak

(a) When this breakthrough pain is at its worst, how would you rate this pain on a scale from 0 to 10, with 0 being 'no pain' and 10 being 'worst possible pain'?

(b) How would you rate the intensity of this breakthrough pain at its worst?

☐ Mild

☐ Moderate

☐ Severe

Q5. Location

Where do you feel this pain? (Please **shade in the entire area** in which you experience this pain)

Q6. Quality

What does the pain feel like? (check √ all that apply)

☐ Throbbing   ☐ Shooting

☐ Stabbing   ☐ Sharp

☐ Cramping   ☐ Gnawing

☐ Hot-Burning   ☐ Aching

☐ Heavy   ☐ Tender

☐ Splitting   ☐ Tiring-Exhausting

☐ Sickening   ☐ Fearful

☐ Punishing-Cruel

☐ Other (please describe):

Q7. Time from onset to peak intensity

When you are awake, on average, how long does it usually take from the time you first feel this pain **until it is at its worst?**

☐ more than 0 and up to 10 minutes

☐ more than 10 and up to 30 minutes

☐ more than 30 minutes

☐ It's hard to say exactly when it started

Q8. Time from onset to end of episode

For those pain episodes that you take breakthrough pain medication, how long does it usually take from the time you take your medication until the pain goes away?

☐ more than 0 and up to 10 minutes

☐ more than 10 and up to 30 minutes

☐ more than 30 minutes

☐ I am not on any breakthrough pain medication

Q9. Cause(s)

Is there anything that triggers this breakthrough pain? (check √ all that apply)

☐ Movement in bed   ☐ Walking

☐ Standing   ☐ Sitting

☐ Coughing   ☐ Vomiting

☐ Having a bowel movement   ☐ Urinating

☐ Swallowing   ☐ Eating

☐ Touching area of skin   ☐ Breathing

☐ It recurs when I feel my scheduled pain medication wearing off

☐ No, nothing in particular triggers this pain

☐ Unsure

☐ Other (please describe):

Q10. Predictability Can you predict when your breakthrough pain will occur?	☐ I can never predict when it will occur ☐ I can rarely predict when it will occur ☐ I can sometimes predict when it will occur ☐ I can often predict when it will occur ☐ I can always predict when it will occur
Q11. General relief Does anything help to relieve or prevent your breakthrough pain? (check √ all that apply)	☐ Moving ☐ Sitting ☐ Rolling over ☐ Lying ☐ Urinating ☐ Having a bowel movement ☐ Passing gas ☐ Burping ☐ Eating ☐ Sleeping ☐ Applying heat ☐ Applying cold ☐ Breathing ☐ Avoiding coughing ☐ Touching/rubbing/squeezing painful area ☐ Use of breakthrough pain medication ☐ Use of scheduled pain medication ☐ Unsure ☐ Other (please describe):
Q12. Relief from breakthrough pain medication In the past *24 hours*, how much relief has your breakthrough pain medication provided for this breakthrough pain?	☐ No relief ☐ Slight relief ☐ Good relief ☐ Very good relief ☐ Complete relief ☐ Not applicable: I haven't taken any breakthrough pain medication in the past 24 hours (skip questions 13-15)
Q13. Satisfaction with breakthrough pain medication In the past *24 hours*, how satisfied have you been with how well your breakthrough pain medication works for this breakthrough pain?	☐ Very satisfied ☐ Moderately satisfied ☐ Slightly satisfied ☐ Neutral ☐ Slightly dissatisfied ☐ Moderately dissatisfied ☐ Very dissatisfied
Q14. Onset of pain relief In the past *24 hours*, on average, how long has it taken for your breakthrough pain medication to *begin* to reduce your breakthrough pain? (Fill in the blank)	____ minutes
Q15. Satisfaction with onset of pain relief In the past *24 hours*, how satisfied have you been with how fast your pain medication *begins* to reduce your breakthrough pain?	☐ Very satisfied ☐ Moderately satisfied ☐ Slightly satisfied ☐ Neutral ☐ Slightly dissatisfied ☐ Moderately dissatisfied ☐ Very dissatisfied

(*Continued*)

TO BE COMPLETED BY PHYSICIAN OR NURSE	
Q1. Etiology of breakthrough pain (check √ all that apply)	Pain related to the site of active cancer
	Pain related to the whole body or systemic effects of the cancer disease process (e.g. muscle spasm or bedsores from debility, pain from shingles, etc.)
	Pain related to anticancer treatment (e.g. side effects of radiotherapy, chemotherapy, surgery)
	Pain caused by a concurrent disorder (e.g. osteoarthritis)
	Unknown or uncertain at this time
Q2. Inferred pathophysiology of breakthrough pain (check √ all that apply)	Somatic nociceptive *List damaged tissues:*
	Visceral nociceptive *List damaged tissues:*
	Neuropathic *List damaged tissues:*
	Unknown or uncertain at this time

References

Bennett M. (2001) The LANSS Pain Scale: the Leeds assessment of neuropathic symptoms and signs. *Pain*, **92**, 147–57.

Caraceni, A., Cherny, N., Fainsinger, R. *et al* (2002) Pain measurement tools and methods in clinical research in palliative care: recommendations of an Expert Working Group of the European Association of Palliative Care. *Journal of Pain and Symptom Management*, **23**, 239–55.

Collins, S.L., Moore, A., McQuay, H.J. (1997) The visual analogue pain intensity scale: what is moderate pain in millimetres? *Pain*, **72**, 95–7.

Daut, R.L., Cleeland, C.S., Flanery, R.C. (1983) Development of the Wisconsin Brief Pain Questionnaire to assess pain in cancer and other diseases. *Pain*, **17**, 197–210.

Davies, A. (2002) The assessment and measurement of physical pain. In Hillier, R., Finlay, I., Miles, A., ed. *The Effective Management of Cancer Pain*, 2nd edn, pp. 23–8. Aesculapius Medical Press, London.

Davies, A.N., Dickman, A., Reid, C., Stevens, A.M., Zeppetella, G. (2009) The management of cancer-related breakthrough pain: recommendations of a task group of the Science Committee of the Association for Palliative Medicine of Great Britain and Ireland. *European Journal of Pain*, **13**, 331–8.

Davies, A. (2010) Breakthrough pain is often poorly controlled in patients with cancer. *Guidelines in Practice*, **13**, 37–40.

de Wit, R., van Dam, F., Abu-Saad, H.H. *et al* (1999) Empirical comparison of commonly used measures to evaluate pain treatment in cancer patients with chronic pain. *Journal of Clinical Oncology*, **17**, 1280–7.

Fishman, B., Pasternak, S., Wallenstein, S.L., Houde, R.W., Holland, J.C., Foley, K.M. (1987) The Memorial Pain Assessment Card: a valid instrument for the evaluation of cancer pain. *Cancer*, **60**, 1151–8.

Foley, K.M. (2004) Acute and chronic cancer pain syndromes. In Doyle, D., Hanks, G., Cherny, N., Calman, K., eds. *Oxford Textbook of Palliative Medicine*, 3rd edn, pp. 298–316. Oxford University Press, Oxford.

Hagen, N.A. (1999) Reproducing a cancer patient's pain on physical examination: bedside provocative maneuvers. *Journal of Pain and Symptom Management*, **18**, 406–11.

Hagen, N.A., Stiles, C., Nekolaichuk, C. *et al* (2009) The Alberta Breakthrough Pain Assessment Tool for cancer patients: a validation study using a Delphi process and patient think-aloud interviews. *Journal of Pain and Symptom Management*, **35**, 136–52.

McQuay, H.J., Moore, R.A. (1998) *An Evidence-based Resource for Pain Relief*. Oxford University Press, Oxford.

Melzack, R. (1975) The McGill Pain Questionnaire: major properties and scoring methods. *Pain*, **1**, 277–99.

Portenoy, R.K., Hagen, N.A. (1990) Breakthrough pain: definition, prevalence and characteristics. *Pain*, **41**, 273–81.

Portenoy, R.K., Payne, D., Jacobsen, P. (1999) Breakthrough pain: characteristics and impact in patients with cancer pain. *Pain*, **81**, 129–34.

Rasmussen, P.V., Sindrup, S.H., Jensen, T.S., Bach, F.W. (2004) Symptoms and signs in patients with suspected neuropathic pain. *Pain*, **110**, 461–9.

Serlin, R.C., Mendoza, T.R., Nakamura, Y., Edwards, K.R., Cleeland, C.S. (1995) When is cancer pain mild, moderate or severe? Grading pain severity by its interference with function. *Pain*, **61**, 277–84.

Shannon, M.M., Ryan, M.A., D'Agostino, N., Brescia, F.J. (1995) Assessment of pain in advanced cancer patients. *Journal of Pain and Symptom Management*, **10**, 274–8.

Trowbridge, R., Dugan, W., Jay, S.J. *et al* (1997) Determining the effectiveness of a clinical-practice intervention in improving the control of pain in outpatients with cancer. *Academic Medicine*, **72**, 798–800.

Twycross, R. (1994) *Pain Relief in Advanced Cancer*. Churchill Livingstone, Edinburgh.

Webber, K., Davies, A.N., Cowie, M.R. (2010) Development of the Breakthrough Pain Assessment Tool (BAT) [Abstract PT016]. In *Proceedings of 13th World Congress on Pain*. 29 August–2 September, Montreal, Canada.

Zeppetella, G., Ribeiro, M.D. (2002) Episodic pain in patients with advanced cancer. *American Journal of Hospice and Palliative Care*, **19**, 267–76.

Chapter 4

General principles of management

> **Key points**
> - Breakthrough pain is not a single entity, but a spectrum of very different entities
> - The treatment of breakthrough pain depends on a variety of pain-related factors
> - This chapter discusses the general principles of the treatment of breakthrough pain
> - The treatment of breakthrough pain depends on the aetiology, pathophysiology and characteristics of the pain
> - The stage of the disease and the performance status of the patient are also important factors.

4.1 Introduction

Breakthrough pain is not a single entity, but a spectrum of very different entities. The optimal management of breakthrough pain depends on a variety of pain-related factors, including the aetiology of the pain (cancer-related, treatment-related, concomitant illness), the pathophysiology of the pain (nociceptive, neuropathic, mixed), and the clinical features of the pain (Davies et al, 2009). Moreover, the management of breakthrough pain depends on a variety of patient-related factors, including the stage of the disease (early, advanced), the performance status of the patient (good, poor), and the personal preferences of the patient.

4.2 Management strategies

The following discussion is based on generic recommendations produced by a Task Group of the Association for Palliative Medicine of Great Britain and Ireland (Davies et al, 2009).

1. **Patients with pain should be assessed for the presence of breakthrough pain (Grade of recommendation – D).**
2. **Patients with breakthrough pain should have this pain specifically assessed (D).**

The assessment of breakthrough pain is discussed in detail in Chapter 3.

3. **The management of breakthrough pain should be individualized (D).**
4. **Consideration should be given to treatment of the underlying cause of the pain (D).**

In most (65–76%) cases, the underlying cause of the pain is a direct effect of the cancer (see Table 1.3) (Portenoy & Hagen, 1990; Portenoy et al, 1999a; Zeppetella et al, 2000). The options for treatment are potentially numerous, with new treatments emerging all the time, and so it is important that there is close liaison with the relevant oncology team. It should be noted that whilst there is good evidence for the efficacy of many oncological treatments in managing background pain, there is relatively little evidence for the efficacy of these treatments in managing breakthrough pain (e.g. conventional radiotherapy). The reason for the lack of evidence relates to a lack of relevant studies, rather than a lack of efficacy per se.

However, there is emerging evidence to suggest certain oncological treatments may indeed be effective in managing certain types of breakthrough pain. For example, Ripamonti et al reported improvements in movement-related/incident pain in 10 (out of 11) patients with bone metastases following treatment with radioactive samarium (Ripamonti et al, 2007a). Similarly, various authors have reported improvements in movement-related/incident pain in patients with bone metastases following treatment with new generation bisphosphonates (Ripamonti et al, 2007b; Galvez et al, 2008).

5. **Consideration should be given to avoidance/treatment of the precipitating factors of the pain (D).**

Avoidance or treatment of precipitating factors should be considered in patients with incident-type breakthrough pain. However, only certain precipitants are amenable to specific interventions (see Table 1.2).

Movement-related/incident pain, secondary to metastatic bone disease, is a common phenomenon. Moreover, studies suggest that this can be the most difficult type of breakthrough pain to manage (Hwang et al, 2003). In some cases, it may be possible to perform surgical stabilization of the relevant bone(s) (Figure 4.1a and b). Alternatively, in other cases, it may be possible to use an orthoptic device to stabilize the relevant bone(s) (Figure 4.2). However, many patients will benefit from strategies to minimize the amount of movement required, such as provision of simple adaptations to their surroundings, and provision of additional practical support with the activities of daily living (Mercadante & Arcuri, 1998).

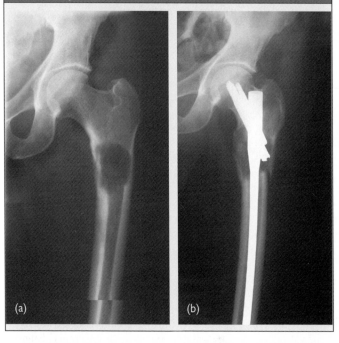

Fig 4.1(a) and (b) Radiographs demonstrating surgical stabilisation of a lytic bone metastasis

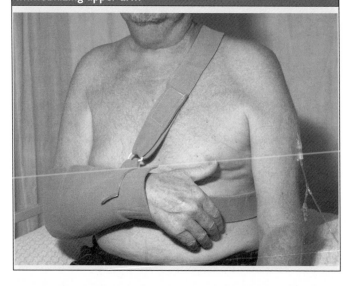

Fig 4.2 Orthotic device (Polysling®) for supporting / immobilizing upper arm

6. **Consideration should be given to modification of the background analgesic regimen/'around the clock medication' (D).**

Modification of the background analgesic regimen has been shown to be a useful approach in managing breakthrough pain (Hwang *et al*, 2003), and may involve one or more of the following treatment strategies:

- Titration of opioid analgesics – titrating the opioid can be effective in reducing the intensity and/or frequency of all types of breakthrough pain (Portenoy, 1997; Mercadante *et al*, 2004). It has been suggested that the dose is initially increased by 25–50% (Portenoy, 1997). However, this strategy is often limited by the existence/development of dose-dependent adverse effects (e.g. sedation) (Portenoy, 1997).

- Switching of opioid analgesics – switching the opioid and/or the route of administration of the opioid can also be effective in reducing the severity of movement-related/incident pain (Kalso *et al*, 1996; Enting *et al*, 2002).

- Addition of 'adjuvant analgesics' – adjuvant analgesics ('co-analgesics') are agents whose primary function is not analgesia, but which provide pain relief in certain circumstances (Lussier & Portenoy, 2004). This strategy can be effective in reducing the impact of specific breakthrough pain syndromes (e.g. antiepileptics for neuropathic pain, antispasmodics for visceral pain).

- Addition of other 'adjuvant drugs' – adjuvant drugs are agents whose function is not analgesia, but which provide relief from the adverse effects of analgesic drugs (or the complications of the pain) (Lussier & Portenoy, 2004). This strategy can be effective in allowing titration of the analgesic drugs, which in turn can be effective in reducing the impact of breakthrough pain (e.g. psychostimulants for opioid-related sedation) (Bruera *et al*, 1992).

Other strategies – in theory, alteration and/or addition of non-opioid analgesic drugs could also lead to improvements in breakthrough pain (e.g. paracetamol, non-steroidal anti-inflammatory drugs).

7. **Opioids are the 'rescue medication' of choice in the management of breakthrough pain episodes (D).**

The cornerstone of the management of breakthrough pain episodes is the use of so-called 'rescue medication'. Rescue medication is taken as required, rather than on a regular basis: in the case of spontaneous pain or non-volitional incident pain the treatment should be taken at the onset of the breakthrough pain; in the case of volitional incident pain or procedural pain the treatment should be taken before the relevant precipitant of the pain. (In the latter scenario, it is important that the rescue medication is taken far enough in advance of the relevant precipitant of the pain).

In most cases the most appropriate rescue medication will be an opioid analgesic, rather than a non-opioid or an adjuvant analgesic. However, opioid preparations will only be effective if the breakthrough pain is an opioid-responsive pain. The decision to use a specific opioid preparation should be based on a combination of the pain characteristics (onset, duration), the product characteristics (pharmacokinetics, pharmacodynamics), the patient's previous response to opioids (efficacy, tolerability), and particularly the patient's preference for an individual preparation.

Opioid rescue medication is discussed in detail in Chapter 5 (oral, rectal and parenteral formulations), Chapter 6 (oral transmucosal formulations), and Chapter 7 (intranasal and intrapulmonary formulations).

8. **The dose of opioid 'rescue medication' should be determined by individual titration (B).**

Traditionally, it has been advised that the dose of opioid rescue medication should be a fixed proportion of the dose of the opioid background medication (Hanks et al, 2001). Data from controlled trials with oral transmucosal fentanyl formulations suggest that there is no relationship between the most effective dose of these preparations and the effective dose of the background opioid medication (Christie et al, 1998; Portenoy et al, 1999b; Coluzzi et al, 2001; Portenoy et al, 2006; Slatkin et al, 2007). Moreover, data from one of these studies suggests that there may be no relationship between the most effective dose of oral morphine for breakthrough pain and the effective dose of the background opioid medication (Coluzzi et al, 2001). It should be noted that the findings in these research studies is supported by the findings in clinical practice (Portenoy & Hagen, 1990; Coluzzi et al, 2001).

9. **Non-pharmacological methods may be useful in the management of breakthrough pain episodes (D).**

Non-pharmacological methods are discussed in detail in Chapter 9.

10. **Non-opioid analgesics may be useful in the management of breakthrough pain episodes (D).**

Non-opioid analgesics are discussed in detail in Chapter 8.

11. **Interventional techniques may be useful in the management of breakthrough pain (D).**

Interventional techniques are discussed in detail in Chapter 9.

12. **Patients with breakthrough pain should have this pain specifically re-assessed (D).**

The re-assessment of breakthrough pain is discussed in detail in Chapter 3.

It should be noted that the Task Group also recommended that patients with difficult-to-manage pain should be referred 'in a timely manner' to a relevant specialist with an interest in breakthrough cancer pain.

Table 4.1 Relieving factors of breakthrough pain in studies applying recognized criteria for breakthrough pain

Study	Relieving factors			Comments
	Medication	Other strate- gies	No relieving factors	
Portenoy & Hagen, 1990	44%	44%	12%	
Portenoy et al, 1999	61%	26%	13%	
Hwang et al, 2003	54%	26%	20%	Data refer to initial assessment (see text).
Davies et al, 2011	57%	46%	12%	16% patients had both medication and 'other strategy' as relieving factors

Table 4.1 shows the relieving factors reported by patients in studies applying standard criteria for the diagnosis of breakthrough pain (Portenoy & Hagen, 1990; Portenoy et al, 1999a; Hwang et al, 2003; Davies et al, 2011). It can be seen that only 44–61% patients reported that their medication relieved breakthrough pain. Nevertheless, Hwang et al have shown that alterations in medication can lead to improvements in breakthrough pain (Hwang et al, 2003). Thus, 54% of patients reported that their medication relieved breakthrough pain at baseline, whilst 83% of patients reported that their medication relieved breakthrough pain after one week of intervention. It should be noted that patients often report more than one relieving factor, e.g. a non-pharmacological intervention and a pharmacological intervention (Portenoy & Hagen, 1990, Davies et al, 2011).

4.3 **Management of end-of-dose failure**

The management of end-of-dose failure involves modification of the background analgesic regimen (Mercadante et al, 2002). The options are:

- Increase the dose of the analgesic – this is the recommended strategy for treating end of dose failure with most opioid analgesics (e.g. morphine, oxycodone) (Hanks et al, 2001). This strategy is invariably effective, although the increase in dosage may lead to an increase in side effects. Indeed, some patients may be unable to tolerate an increase in dosage (Simmonds, 1999)

- Increase the frequency of the analgesic – this is a recommended strategy for treating end of dose failure with transdermal fentanyl (see below) (Breitbart et al, 2000). This strategy has also been used for treating end-of-dose failure with other opioids (Hanks et al, 2001). Nevertheless, this strategy is not recommended for treating end-of-dose failure with other opioids (Hanks et al, 2001).

  In most patients, the duration of action of transdermal fentanyl is 72hr. Nevertheless, in some (3–43%) patients, the duration of action of transdermal fentanyl is somewhere between 48–72hr (Payne et al, 1995; Grond et al, 1997). It has been recommended that patients who are pain controlled for 48hr, but who require breakthrough medication between 48–72hr, should replace their patch every 48hr rather than every 72hr (and rather than increasing the dose of the patch) (Breitbart et al, 2000)

- Provision of additional analgesic drugs/other pain relief methods.

It should be noted that many experts believe that end-of-dose failure is not a subtype of breakthrough pain (see Chapter 1) (Davies et al, 2009).

4.4 **Other issues**

4.4.1 **Prescription of rescue medication**

Studies suggest that patients are frequently not prescribed rescue medication. For example, Ferrell et al reported that 27% patients in their study had not been prescribed rescue medication (Ferrell et al, 1999). Other authors have reported even higher levels of non-prescription (i.e. 38–57%) (Weber & Huber, 1999; Zeppetella et al, 2000b; Lawrie et al, 2003). Ferrell et al also reported that patients that had been prescribed rescue medication in their study, had had inappropriate limitations imposed on the frequency of use of the rescue medication (Ferrell et al, 1999). Thus, only 29% patients were told that they could use the rescue medication the recommended 1–2 hrly (if required) (Ferrell et al, 1999).

4.4.2 **Adherence with rescue medication**

Non-adherence with prescribed medication appears to be common amongst patients with cancer. For example, Zeppetella et al reported that 44% of homecare patients were not taking their medication as prescribed (Zeppetella, 1999). In particular, patients were not taking their analgesics as prescribed (i.e. non-opioids, opioids).

Ferrell et al reported that only 3% patients were taking their rescue medication as prescribed (Ferrell et al, 1999). Thus, 96% patients were taking too low a dose, 3% patients were taking the prescribed

Table 4.2 Reasons for not always taking rescue medication (Davies et al, 2008)

Reasons for not taking break-through medication	Primary reason (n = 63)	Other reasons* (n = 63)	Comments
Pain is not always intense/severe	25	21	
Pain improves before medication starts to work	3	18	
Medication isn't effective	1	4	
Restrictions on use of medication	1	3	The restrictions on use of medication involved either the total number of doses of breakthrough medication, or the time interval between doses of breakthrough medication.
Side effects of medication	7	10	
Concerns about side effects of medication	9	4	
Concerns about over dosage	3	9	
Concerns about tolerance	3	10	
Concerns about addiction	2	11	
Other reasons	9	8	The other reasons involved dislike of medication (7 patients); polypharmacy (3 patients); use of different strategies in different scenarios (2 patients); use of pain as a marker of disease status (1 patient); fatigue (1 patient); depression (1 patient); no specific reason (2 patients).

*Subjects could have more than one reason.

dose, and 1% patients were taking too high a dose. Indeed, the mean dose taken was only 21% of the dose prescribed.

Similarly, Davies et al reported that only 18.5% patients used their rescue medication every time they experienced breakthrough pain (Davies et al, 2008). The patients' reasons for not always taking rescue medication were varied (Table 4.2), whilst the patients' criteria for actually taking rescue medication were also varied (e.g. duration of pain, intensity of pain).

Interestingly, Gómez-Batiste et al reported that the use of rescue medication depends on the type of breakthrough pain (Gómez-Batiste et al, 2002). Thus, patients with incident pain were less likely to use breakthrough medication than patients with spontaneous pain. The most likely reason for this phenomenon is that incident pain tends to be of shorter duration than spontaneous pain, and so is less likely to respond to rescue medication.

4.4.3 Acceptability of rescue medication

One of the factors that may affect adherence is the acceptability of the rescue medication. Table 4.3 shows the acceptability of different routes of administration to palliative care patients if the pain was rated as 'mild to moderate' (Walker et al, 2003). Similarly, Table 4.4 shows the acceptability of these routes of administration to palliative care patients if the pain was rated as 'severe' (Walker et al, 2003). (It should be noted that patients were informed that the onset of pain relief was 5 min for the IV route; 10 min for the nasal, sublingual, transmucosal, inhaled, SC and IM routes; and 30 min for the oral and rectal routes). It can be seen that the acceptability of a route was somewhat dependent on the severity of the pain, i.e. the more severe the pain the more likely the patient will accept an invasive route of administration.

In contrast, Davies et al did not find that the acceptability of a route was associated with the actual severity of the pain (Davies et al, 2011). However, they did find that the acceptability of a route was associated with previous use of the route (e.g. patients with experience of subcutaneous route were more likely to consider using this route than patients without experience of subcutaneous route), and that there were certain cultural differences (e.g. Danish patients were less likely to consider using the oral transmucosal route than British patients) and gender differences (e.g. male patients were more likely to consider using the intranasal route than female patients). Table 4.5 shows the reasons given for not wanting to use different routes of administration.

Table 4.3 Acceptability of different routes of administration of breakthrough medication for mild-to-moderate pain (Walker et al, 2003)

Route	Acceptability of route for mild to moderate pain			Reasons for unacceptability
	Yes (%)	Possibly (%)	No (%)	
Oral	97	1	2	Slow onset of action
Rectal	24	19	57	Dignity, previous bad experience, localized pain/disease, difficult to administer, unpleasant/uncomfortable, 'inappropriate for level of pain'
Nasal	50	18	32	Localized pain/disease, difficult to administer, catches back of throat, fear of bad taste/nausea, unpleasant/uncomfortable, unfamiliar/dislike idea
Sublingual	63	19	18	Previous bad experience, fear of bad taste/nausea, unfamiliar/dislike idea
Transmucosal	44	21	35	Fear of bad taste/nausea, 'childlike', unfamiliar/dislike idea, risk of children taking drug
Inhaled	60	19	21	Previous bad experience, localized pain/disease, difficult to administer, fear of bad taste/nausea, unfamiliar/dislike idea
Subcutaneous	52	20	28	'Inappropriate for level of pain', dislike of injections
Intramuscular	33	22	45	'Inappropriate for level of pain', dislike of injections
Intravenous	38	23	39	Previous bad experience, 'inappropriate for level of pain', dislike of injections

Table 4.4 Acceptability of different routes of administration of breakthrough medication for severe pain (Walker et al, 2003)

Route	Acceptability of route for severe pain			Reasons for unacceptability
	Yes (%)	Possibly (%)	No (%)	
Oral	88	4	8	Slow onset of action
Rectal	48	10	42	Slow onset of action, dignity, previous bad experience, localized pain/disease, difficult to administer, unpleasant/uncomfortable
Nasal	68	14	18	Localized pain/disease, difficult to administer, catches back of throat, fear of bad taste/nausea, unfamiliar/dislike idea
Sublingual	75	11	14	Slow onset of action, previous bad experience, fear of bad taste/nausea, unfamiliar/dislike idea
Transmucosal	63	12	25	Localized pain/disease, fear of bad taste/nausea, 'childlike', unfamiliar/dislike idea
Inhaled	75	9	16	Previous bad experience, localized pain/disease, difficult to administer, fear of bad taste/nausea, unfamiliar/dislike idea
Subcutaneous	87	8	5	Dislike of injections
Intramuscular	76	12	12	Dislike of injections
Intravenous	83	8	9	Previous bad experience, dislike of injections

Table 4.5 Reasons for not wanting to use different routes of administration (Davies *et al*, 2011) (Reproduced with permission from John Wiley & Sons. © 2011).

Route of delivery	Reasons for not wanting to use route of delivery	Number positive responses*	Number 'main reason' responses
Oral transmucosal (n = 29)	Current/previous problems with mouth	9	9
	'I don't like idea of such a product'	11	8
	Previous bad experience	1	0
	Concerns about effectiveness	3	3
	Concerns about side effects	2	1
	Concerns about addiction	1	1
	Other reasons	5	4
	Not stated	1	3
Intranasal (n = 82)	Current/previous problems with nose	20	13
	'I don't like idea of such a product'	52	38
	Previous bad experience	5	4
	Concerns about effectiveness	11	5
	Concerns about side effects	8	2
	Concerns about addiction	7	4
	Other reasons	6	5
	Not stated	6	11

Intrapulmonary (n = 70)	Current/previous problems with lungs	17	12
	'I don't like idea of such a product'	**44**	**33**
	Previous bad experience	2	0
	Concerns about effectiveness	14	8
	Concerns about side effects	8	4
	Concerns about addiction	4	1
	Other reasons	7	7
	Not stated	3	5
Subcutaneous (n = 58)	Current/previous problems with skin	9	5
	'I don't like idea of such a product'	**36**	**28**
	Previous bad experience	5	2
	Concerns about effectiveness	4	0
	Concerns about side effects	6	1
	Concerns about addiction	2	2
	Other reasons	11	11
	Not stated	7	9

*Patient could give any / all reasons.

References

Breitbart, W., Chandler, S., Eagel, B. *et al* (2000) An alternative algorithm for dosing transdermal fentanyl for cancer-related pain. *Oncology* (Huntington), **14**, 695–705.

Bruera, E., Fainsinger, R., MacEachern, T., Hanson, J. (1992) The use of methylphenidate in patients with incident cancer pain receiving regular opiates. A preliminary report. *Pain*, **50**, 75–7.

Christie, J.M., Simmonds, M., Patt, R. *et al* (1998) Dose-titration, multicenter study of oral transmucosal fentanyl citrate for the treatment of breakthrough pain in cancer patients using transdermal fentanyl for persistent pain. *Journal of Clinical Oncology*, **16**, 3238–45.

Coluzzi, P.H., Schwartzberg, L., Conroy, Jr J.D. *et al* (2001) Breakthrough cancer pain: a randomized trial comparing oral transmucosal fentanyl citrate (OTFC) and morphine sulfate immediate release (MSIR). *Pain*, **91**, 123–30.

Davies, A.N., Vriens, J., Kennett, A., McTaggart, M. (2008) An observational study of oncology patients' utilisation of breakthrough pain medication. *Journal of Pain and Symptom Management*, **35**, 406–11.

Davies, A.N., Dickman, A., Reid, C., Stevens, A.M., Zeppetella, G. (2009) The management of cancer-related breakthrough pain: recommendations of a task group of the Science Committee of the Association for Palliative Medicine of Great Britain and Ireland. *European Journal of Pain*, **13**, 331–8.

Davies, A., Zeppetella, G., Andersen, S. *et al* (2011) Multi-centre European study of breakthrough cancer pain: pain characteristics and patient perceptions of current and potential management strategies. *European Journal of Pain*, **15**, 756–63.

Enting, R.H., Oldenmenger, W.H., van der Rijt, C.C. *et al* (2002) A prospective study evaluating the response of patients with unrelieved cancer pain to parenteral opioids. *Cancer*, **94**, 3049–56.

Ferrell, B.R., Juarez, G., Borneman, T. (1999) Use of routine and breakthrough analgesia in home care. *Oncology Nursing Forum*, **26**, 1655–61.

Fine, P.G., Busch, M.A. (1998) Characterization of breakthrough pain by hospice patients and their caregivers. *Journal of Pain and Symptom Management*, **16**, 179–83.

Galvez, R., Ribera, V., Gonzalez-Escalada, J.R. *et al* (2008) Analgesic efficacy of zoledronic acid and its effect on functional status of prostate cancer patients. *Patient Preference and Adherence*, **2**, 215–24.

Gómez-Batiste, X., Madrid, F., Moreno, F. *et al* (2002) Breakthrough cancer pain: prevalence and characteristics in patients in Catalonia, Spain. *Journal of Pain and Symptom Management*, **24**, 45–52.

Grond, S., Zech, D., Lehmann, K.A., Radbruch, L., Breitenbach, H., Hertel, D. (1997) Transdermal fentanyl in the long-term treatment of cancer pain: a prospective study of 50 patients with advanced cancer of the gastrointestinal tract or the head and neck region. *Pain*, **69**, 191–8.

Hanks, G.W., de Conno, F., Cherny, N. *et al* (2001) Morphine and alternative opioids in cancer pain: the EAPC recommendations. *British Journal of Cancer*, **84**, 587–93.

Hwang, S.S., Chang, V.T., Kasimis, B. (2003) Cancer breakthrough pain characteristics and responses to treatment at a VA medical center. *Pain*, **101**, 55–64.

Kalso, E., Heiskanen, T., Rantio, M., Rosenberg, P.H., Vainio, A. (1996) Epidural and subcutaneous morphine in the management of cancer pain: a double-blind cross-over study. *Pain*, **67**, 443–9.

Lawrie, I., Lloyd-Williams, M., Waterhouse, E. (2003) Breakthrough strong opioid analgesia prescription in patients using transdermal fentanyl admitted to a hospice. *American Journal of Hospice and Palliative Care*, **20**, 229–30.

Lussier, D., Portenoy, R.K. (2004) Adjuvant analgesics in pain management. In Doyle, D., Hanks, G., Cherny, N., Calman, K., ed. *Oxford Textbook of Palliative Medicine*, 3rd edn, pp. 349–78. Oxford University Press, Oxford.

Mercadante, S., Arcuri, E. (1998) Breakthrough pain in cancer patients: pathophysiology and treatment. *Cancer Treatment Reviews*, **24**, 425–32.

Mercadante, S., Radbruch, L., Caraceni, A. *et al* (2002) Episodic (breakthrough) pain. Consensus conference of an Expert Working Group of the European Association for Palliative Care. *Cancer*, **94**, 832–9.

Mercadante, S., Villari, P., Ferrera, P., Casuccio, A. (2004) Optimization of opioid therapy for preventing incident pain associated with bone metastases. *Journal of Pain and Symptom Management*, **28**, 505–10.

Payne, R., Chandler, S., Einhaus, M. (1995) Guidelines for the clinical use of transdermal fentanyl. *Anti-Cancer Drugs*, **6**(3), 50–3.

Portenoy, R.K., Hagen, N.A. (1990) Breakthrough pain: definition, prevalence and characteristics. *Pain*, **41**, 273–81.

Portenoy, R.K. (1997) Treatment of temporal variations in chronic cancer pain. *Seminars in Oncology*, **5**, S16–7.12.

Portenoy, R.K., Payne, D., Jacobsen, P. (1999a) Breakthrough pain: characteristics and impact in patients with cancer pain. *Pain*, **81**, 129–34.

Portenoy, R.K., Payne, R., Coluzzi, P. *et al* (1999b) Oral transmucosal fentanyl citrate (OTFC) for the treatment of breakthrough pain in cancer patients: a controlled dose titration study. *Pain*, **79**, 303–12.

Portenoy, R.K., Taylor, D., Messina, J., Tremmel, L. (2006) A randomized, placebo-controlled study of fentanyl buccal tablet for breakthrough pain in opioid-treated patients with cancer. *Clinical Journal of Pain*, **22**, 805–11.

Ripamonti, C., Fagnoni, E., Campa, T., Seregni, E., Maccauro, M., Bombardieri, E. (2007a) Incident pain and analgesic consumption decrease after samarium infusion: a pilot study. *Supportive Care in Cancer*, **15**, 339–42.

Ripamonti, C., Fagnoni, E., Campa, T. *et al* (2007b) Decreases in pain at rest and movement-related pain during zoledronic acid treatment in patients with bone metastases due to breast or prostate cancer: a pilot study. *Supportive Care in Cancer*, **15**, 1177–84.

Simmonds, M.A. (1999) Management of breakthrough pain due to cancer. *Oncology* (Huntington), **13**, 1103–8.

Slatkin, N.E., Xie, F., Messina, J., Segal, T.J. (2007) Fentanyl buccal tablet for relief of breakthrough pain in opioid-tolerant patients with cancer-related chronic pain. *Journal of Supportive Oncology*, **5**, 327–34.

Walker, G., Wilcock, A., Manderson, C., Weller, R., Crosby, V. (2003) The acceptability of different routes of administration of analgesia for break-through pain. *Palliative Medicine*, **17**, 219–21.

Weber, M., Huber, C. (1999) Documentation of severe pain, opioid doses, and opioid-related side effects in outpatients with cancer: a retrospective study. *Journal of Pain and Symptom Management*, **17**, 49–54.

Zeppetella G (1999) How do terminally ill patients at home take their medi-cation? *Palliative Medicine*, **13**, 469–75.

Zeppetella, G., O'Doherty, C.A., Collins, S. (2000) Prevalence and character-istics of breakthrough pain in cancer patients admitted to a hospice. *Journal of Pain and Symptom Management*, **20**, 87–92.

Chapter 5

Oral and parenteral opioids

Key points

- The oral route may not be suitable for many patients with breakthrough pain
- The pharmacokinetic profile of many orally delivered drugs does not mirror breakthrough pain characteristics, resulting in partially effective treatment and/or troublesome adverse effects
- Intravenous/subcutaneous opioids provide rapid onset of analgesia, but are not practical in the community setting.

5.1 Introduction

As discussed in Chapter 4, the cornerstone of the management of breakthrough pain episodes is the use of so-called 'rescue medication' (Davies et al, 2009). Rescue medication is taken as required, rather than on a regular basis: in the case of spontaneous pain or non-volitional incident pain the treatment should be taken at the onset of the breakthrough pain; in the case of volitional incident pain or procedural pain the treatment should be taken before the relevant precipitant of the pain. (In the latter scenario, it is important that the rescue medication is taken far enough in advance of the relevant precipitant of the pain.)

In most cases the most appropriate rescue medication will be an opioid analgesic, rather than a non-opioid or an adjuvant analgesic. However, opioid preparations will only be effective if the breakthrough pain is an opioid-responsive pain. The decision to use a specific opioid preparation should be based on a combination of the pain characteristics (onset, duration), the product characteristics (pharmacokinetics, pharmacodynamics), the patient's previous response to opioids (efficacy, tolerability), and particularly the patient's preference for an individual preparation. This chapter will discuss the use of oral, rectal, and parenteral opioids as rescue medication.

5.2 **Oral opioids**

5.2.1 **Introduction to oral opioids**

The World Health Organization recommends the oral route for treating cancer pain (the concept of 'by mouth') (WHO, 1996). However, although the oral route is generally effective in the management of background pain, it is often less effective in the management of breakthrough pain. Indeed, a Task Group of the Association for Palliative Medicine of Great Britain and Ireland (APM) noted that 'the pharmacoknetic/pharmacodynamic profiles of oral opioids do not tend to mirror the temporal characteristics of most breakthrough pain episodes', and concluded that 'oral opioids are not the optimal rescue medication for most breakthrough pain episodes' (Davies *et al*, 2009).

5.2.2 **Clinical data**

The pharmacodynamic profiles of selective normal-release ('immediate-release') opioids for moderate-to-severe pain ('strong opioids') are shown in Table 5.1. The relatively slow onset of action/time to peak effect limits their efficacy in managing breakthrough cancer pain episodes, whilst the relatively long duration of action may have a negative impact in terms of adverse effects (Figure 5.1).

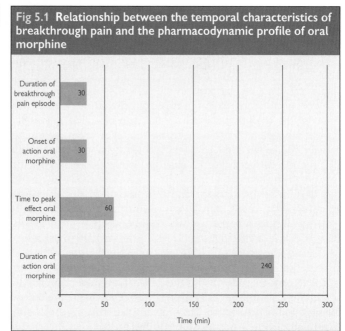

Fig 5.1 **Relationship between the temporal characteristics of breakthrough pain and the pharmacodynamic profile of oral morphine**

Table 5.1 Basic clinical data for opioids for moderate-to-severe pain available in the United Kingdom (Thompson, 1990; Leow et al, 1992, Twycross et al, 1998; Twycross et al, 2002)

Drug	Onset of action	Time to peak effect	Duration of action
Morphine	20–30 min	60–90 min	3–6 hr
Hydromorphone	30 min	No data available	4–5 hr
Methadone	30 min	30–120 min	4–5 hr (single dose)
Oxycodone	20–30 min	120 min	4–6 hr

Zeppetella studied the time to 'meaningful pain relief' after treatment with oral morphine, oral oxycodone, oral hydromorphone, oral methadone and oral transmucosal fentanyl citrate in patients with breakthrough cancer pain (Zeppetella, 2008). The average time to meaningful pain relief was 31 min (range 5–75 min), and there was no difference found amongst the various oral opioids (Figure 5.2).

Coluzzi et al reported that morphine capsules produced 'moderate' pain relief by 60 min post dose, although there was a clinically

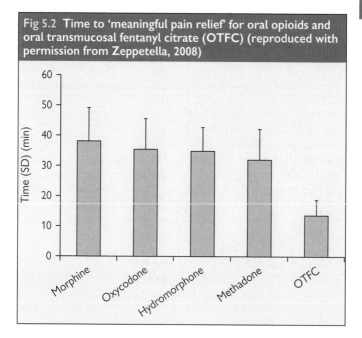

Fig 5.2 Time to 'meaningful pain relief' for oral opioids and oral transmucosal fentanyl citrate (OTFC) (reproduced with permission from Zeppetella, 2008)

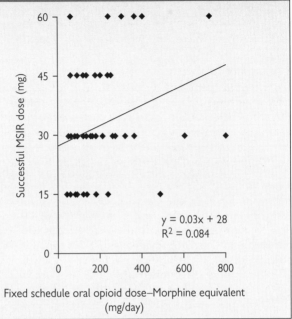

Fig 5.3 Relationship between successful dose of break-through oral morphine ('MSIR') and background dose of oral opioid (reproduced with permission from **Coluzzi** *et al*, 2001)

$y = 0.03x + 28$
$R^2 = 0.084$

Fixed schedule oral opioid dose–Morphine equivalent (mg/day)

significant improvement in pain intensity difference at 30 min post dose (Coluzzi *et al*, 2001). Interestingly, the authors also reported no relationship between the effective dose of the morphine capsules and the dose of the background opioid analgesic (Figure 5.3).

Recently, a novel effervescent morphine tablet was reported to have a faster onset of action than a conventional (non-effervescent) morphine tablet (Freye *et al*, 2007); the mean onset of 'sufficient pain relief' was 13 min (+/- 5.6 min) for the novel morphine tablet and 27 min (+/- 4.4 min) for the conventional morphine tablet. The authors also reported no relationship between the effective dose of the novel morphine tablet and the dose of the background opioid analgesic.

Nevertheless, oral opioids do have a role in the management of breakthrough pain (Davies *et al*, 2009). They may be useful in the management of breakthrough pain episodes lasting for more than 60 min, and may be considered in the pre-emptive management of volitional incident pain or procedural pain. However, if oral opioids are used in the latter scenario, then they need to be taken at least 30 min before the relevant precipitant of the pain.

5.2.3 **Other issues**

5.2.3.1 Acceptability of route

In a survey looking at the acceptability of different routes of administration for rescue medication, 97% patients stated that the oral route was acceptable for 'mild-to-moderate pain', whilst 88% patients stated that the oral route was acceptable for 'severe pain' (see Tables 4.2 and 4.3) (Walker *et al*, 2003).

5.2.3.2 Drug formulation

There are a number of different formulations of oral opioids for moderate-to-severe pain. The choice of preparation depends on a number of patient-related factors (e.g. patient preference, presence of dysphagia, presence of enteral feeding tube), and a number of drug-related factors (e.g. taste, alcohol content, sucrose content). There is little or no evidence that the formulation of the opioid affects the clinical/pharmacokinetic profile of the opioid (Figure 5.4) (Collins *et al*, 1998).

5.2.3.3 Drug dose

The 'correct' dose of rescue medication is the dose that provides maximal analgesia with minimal side effects (Zeppetella & Ribeiro, 2002). An Expert Working Group of the European Association for Palliative Care has recommended using 1/6 (~ 17%) of the daily dose of background opioid analgesia (Hanks *et al*, 2001). However, the Expert Working Group added that 'it may be that the optimal dose for breakthrough pain can only be determined by titration' (Hanks *et al*, 2001). Other authorities have recommended using between

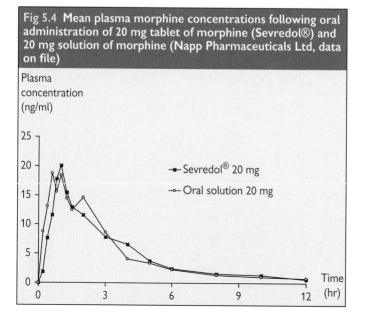

Fig 5.4 Mean plasma morphine concentrations following oral administration of 20 mg tablet of morphine (Sevredol®) and 20 mg solution of morphine (Napp Pharmaceuticals Ltd, data on file)

5–15% of daily dose of background opioid analgesia (Cherny & Portenoy, 1993).

The Task Group of the APM recommended that 'the dose of 'rescue medication' should be determined by individual titration' (Davies *et al*, 2009). Hence, on the basis of the above, it would seem reasonable to initially prescribe 1/6 of the daily dose of background opioid analgesia, and then to titrate the dose upwards/downwards according to the response achieved. Thus, if the pain is not relieved, and side effects are not troublesome, then the dose should be titrated upwards. In contrast, if the pain is relieved, but side effects are troublesome, then the dose should be titrated downwards.

5.2.3.4 Drug costs
The oral route is considered to be relatively cost-effective (Patt & Ellison, 1998). However, although oral opioids are relatively inexpensive to purchase, they will only be truly cost-effective if they actually relieve the breakthrough pain (and impact on the financial burden of breakthrough pain) (Fortner *et al*,2002; Fortner *et al*, 2003).

5.3 **Rectal opioids**

5.3.1 **Introduction to rectal opioids**
The rectal administration of opioids is well established, although is now uncommon in day-to-day clinical practice.

5.3.2 **Clinical data**
The rectal route has been suggested as being suitable for the treatment of breakthrough pain, although there appears to be no specific studies of the use of the rectal route for the treatment of breakthrough pain (Mercadante *et al*, 2002).

5.3.3 **Other issues**
In the aforementioned survey looking at the acceptability of different routes of administration for breakthrough medication, only 24% patients stated that the rectal route was acceptable for 'mild-to-moderate pain', whilst only 48% patients stated that the rectal route was acceptable for 'severe pain' (see Tables 4.2 and 4.3) (Walker *et al*, 2003). A variety of different reasons were given for not wanting to use this route of administration (see Table 4.2).

5.4 **Intravenous opioids**

5.4.1 **Introduction to intravenous opioids**
The intravenous route of administration is primarily used in secondary care settings, especially when a rapid analgesic effect is required,

but also when other routes of administration are unavailable/inappropriate.

The intravenous route is associated with a 100% bioavailability (by definition), and a very rapid onset of action (~ 5 min).

5.4.2 Clinical data

Mercadante and colleagues have published a number of reports of the use of fixed doses of intravenous morphine to treat breakthrough pain episodes (Mercadante *et al*, 2004; Mercadante *et al*, 2006; Mercadante *et al*, 2007; Mercadante *et al*, 2008; Mercadante *et al*, 2010). Intravenous morphine was found to be effective, with most patients achieving clinically meaningful pain relief within 15 min. Moreover, intravenous morphine was found to be well tolerated, and safe to use (in the inpatient setting).

A number of authors have reported the successful use of intravenous opioid patient controlled analgesia (PCA) in both secondary care and in the community setting (Swanson *et al*, 1989; Wagner *et al*, 1989).

5.4.3 Other issues

Intravenous administration has low acceptability when pain is mild-to-moderate in intensity (38% acceptability), but has a much higher acceptability when pain is severe in intensity (83% acceptability) (Walker *et al*, 2003). The main objections to the use of this route are dislike of injections, and previous bad experiences with this route.

5.5 **Subcutaneous opioids**

5.5.1 **Introduction to subcutaneous opioids**

The subcutaneous route is associated with a relatively high bioavailability, and a relatively rapid onset of action (~ 10 min). For example, the bioavailability of subcutaneous morphine is 80–100% (lower for bolus doses, higher for continuous infusions) (Stuart-Harris *et al*, 2000).

5.5.2 **Clinical data**

Enting *et al* reported on the use of various subcutaneous opioids to treat breakthrough pain (e.g. hydromorphone, morphine, sufentanil) (Enting *et al*, 2005): the opioids were delivered using a 'pain pen', which was in fact a modified insulin pen. The authors reported that 84% patients rated the overall efficacy as 'good', and commented that the onset of action was 5–10 min. (Sufentanil is not available in the UK).

A number of authors have again reported the successful use of subcutaneous patient controlled analgesia (PCA) in both secondary care and in the community setting (Swanson *et al*, 1989; Wagner *et al*, 1989).

5.5.3 **Other issues**

Subcutaneous administration has reasonable acceptability when pain is mild-to-moderate in intensity (52% acceptability), but has a much higher acceptability when pain is severe in intensity (87% acceptability) (Walker *et al*, 2003). The main objection to the use of this route was dislike of injections.

5.6 **Intramuscular opioids**

5.6.1 **Introduction to intramuscular opioids**

The intramuscular route is again associated with a relatively high bioavailability, and a relatively rapid onset of action (~ 10 min).

5.6.2 **Clinical data**

It appears that there are no studies of the use of intramuscular opioids to treat breakthrough pain episodes. Moreover, the intramuscular route of administration is not recommended for the treatment of breakthrough pain, because of the discomfort associated with intramuscular injection (Mercadante *et al*, 2002).

5.6.3 **Other issues**

The intramuscular route of administration is not acceptable to many patients, because of their dislike for injections (and particularly intramuscular injections) (see Tables 4.2 and 4.3) (Walker *et al*, 2003).

60

References

Cherny, N.I., Portenoy, R.K. (1993) Cancer pain management. Current strategy. *Cancer*, 72(11), 3393–415.

Collins, S.L., Faura, C.C., Moore, A., McQuay, H.J. (1998) Peak plasma concentrations after oral morphine: a systematic review. *Journal of Pain and Symptom Management*, **16**, 388–402.

Coluzzi, P.H., Schwartzberg, L., Conroy Jr, J.D. *et al* (2001) Breakthrough cancer pain: a randomized trial comparing oral transmucosal fentanyl citrate (OTFC) and morphine sulfate immediate release (MSIR). *Pain*, **91**, 123–30.

Davies, A.N., Dickman, A., Reid, C., Stevens, A.M., Zeppetella, G. (2009) The management of cancer-related breakthrough pain: recommendations of a task group of the Science Committee of the Association for Palliative Medicine of Great Britain and Ireland. *European Journal of Pain*, **13**, 331–8.

Enting, R.H., Mucchiano, C., Oldenmenger, W.H. *et al* (2005) The 'pain pen' for breakthrough cancer pain: a promising treatment. *Journal of Pain and Symptom Management*, **29**, 213–17.

Fortner, B.V., Demarco, G., Irving, G. *et al* (2003) Description and predictors of direct and indirect costs of pain reported by cancer patients. *Journal of Pain and Symptom Management*, **25**, 9–18.

Fortner, B.V., Okon, T.A., Portenoy, R.K. (2002) A survey of pain-related hospitalizations, emergency department visits, and physician office visits reported by cancer patients with and without history of breakthrough pain. *Journal of Pain*, **3**, 38–44.

Freye, E., Levy, J.V., Braun, D. (2007) Effervescent morphine results in faster relief of breakthrough pain in patients compared to immediate release morphine sulfate tablet. *Pain Practice*, **7**, 324–31.

Hanks, G.W., de Conno, F., Cherny, N. *et al* (2001) Morphine and alternative opioids in cancer pain: the EAPC recommendations. *British Journal of Cancer*, **84**, 587–93.

Leow, K.P., Smith, M.T., Williams, B., Cramond, T. (1992) Single-dose and steady-state pharmacokinetics and pharmacodynamics of oxycodone in patients with cancer. *Clinical Pharmacology and Therapeutics*, **52**, 487–95.

Mercadante, S., Radbruch, L., Caraceni, A. *et al* (2002) Episodic (breakthrough) pain. Consensus conference of an Expert Working Group of the European Association for Palliative Care. *Cancer*, **94**, 832–9.

Mercadante, S., Villari, P., Ferrera, P., Bianchi, M., Casuccio, A. (2004) Safety and effectiveness of intravenous morphine for episodic (breakthrough) pain using a fixed ratio with the oral daily morphine dose. *Journal of Pain and Symptom Management*, **27**, 352–9.

Mercadante, S., Villari, P., Ferrera, P., Porzio, G., Aielli, F., Verna, L. *et al* (2006). Safety and effectiveness of intravenous morphine for episodic breakthrough pain in patients receiving transdermal buprenorphine. *Journal of Pain and Symptom Management*, **32**, 175–9.

Mercadante, S., Villari, P., Ferrara, P., Casuccio, A., Mangione, S., Intravaia, G. (2007) Transmucosal fentanyl vs intravenous morphine in doses proportional to basal opioid regimen for episodic-breakthrough pain. *British Journal of Cancer*, **96**, 1828–33.

Mercadante, S., Intravaia, G., Villari, P., Ferrera, P., Riina, S., Mangione, S. (2008) Intravenous morphine for breakthrough (episodic-) pain in an acute palliative care unit: a confirmatory study. *Journal of Pain and Symptom Management*, **35**, 307–13.

Mercadante, S., Villari, P., Ferrara, P., Mangione, S., Casuccio, A. (2010) The use of opioids for breakthrough pain in acute palliative care unit by using doses proportional to opioid basal regimen. *Clinical Journal of Pain*, **26**, 306–9.

Patt, R.B., Ellison, N.M. (1998) Breakthrough pain in cancer patients: characteristics, prevalence, and treatment. *Oncology* (Huntington), **12**, 1035–52.

Stuart-Harris, R., Joel, S.P., McDonald, P., Currow, D., Slevin, M.L. (2000) The pharmacokinetics of morphine and morphine glucuronide metabolites after subcutaneous bolus injection and subcutaneous infusion of morphine. *British Journal of Clinical Pharmacology*, **49**, 207–14.

Swanson, G., Smith, J., Bulich, R., New, P., Shiffman, R. (1989) Patient-controlled analgesia for chronic cancer pain in the ambulatory setting: a report of 117 patients. *Journal of Clinical Oncology*, **7**, 1903–8.

Thompson, J.W. (1990) Clinical pharmacology of opioid agonists and partial agonists. In Doyle, D., ed. *Opioids in the Treatment of Cancer Pain*. pp. 17–38. Royal Society of Medicine Services Ltd, London.

Twycross, R., Wilcock, A., Thorp, S. (1998) *Palliative Care Formulary*. Radcliffe Medical Press Ltd, Abingdon.

Twycross, R., Wilcock, A., Charlesworth, S., Dickman, A. (2002) *Palliative Care Formulary*, 2nd edn. Radcliffe Medical Press, Abingdon.

Wagner, J.C., Souders, G.D., Coffman, L.K., Horvath, J.L. (1989) Management of chronic cancer pain using a computerized ambulatory patient-controlled analgesia pump. *Hospital Pharmacy*, **24**, 639–44.

Walker, G., Wilcock, A., Manderson, C., Weller, R., Crosby, V. (2003) The acceptability of different routes of administration of analgesia for breakthrough pain. *Palliative Medicine*, **17**, 219–21.

World Health Organization (1996) *Cancer Pain Relief*, 2nd edn. World Health Organization, Geneva.

Zeppetella, G. (2008) Opioids for cancer breakthrough pain: a pilot study reporting patient assessment of time to meaningful pain relief. *Journal of Pain and Symptom Management*, **35**, 563–7.

Zeppetella, G., Ribeiro, M.D. (2002) Episodic pain in patients with advanced cancer. *American Journal of Hospice and Palliative Care*, **19**, 267–76.

Chapter 6

Oral transmucosal opioids

Key points
• The oral transmucosal routes are buccal and sublingual
• Oral transmucosal routes are non-invasive, convenient for patients and for healthcare professionals, with a potentially fast onset of action
• A number of fentanyl-based formulations are commercially available.

6.1 Introduction

As discussed in Chapter 5, the oral route of administration is not suitable for many patients with breakthrough cancer pain. Indeed, alternative routes of administration have become increasingly important in the management of this phenomenon. This chapter will focus on the role of the oral transmucosal routes of administration (i.e. buccal route, sublingual route).

6.2 Oral mucosa

The oral mucosa refers to the lining of the oral cavity. It is composed of an outer layer of stratified squamous epithelium, below which lies the basement membrane, and then the lamina propria (connective tissue layer). The total surface area of the oral mucosa is ~ 200 cm^2, which is relatively small compared to the gastrointestinal tract ($\sim$350 000 cm^2) (Zhang et al, 2002). The lamina propria is highly vascularized, and drugs diffusing into the oral mucosa have access to the systemic circulation via its capillaries and venous drainage (internal jugular vein). The rate of blood flow through the oral mucosa is substantial; it is 0.97 ml/min/cm^2 in the sublingual mucosa and 2.4 ml/min/cm^2 in the buccal mucosa. The oral mucosa is covered by a layer of saliva, which is secreted by the three pairs of major salivary glands (parotid, submandibular, sublingual), and the hundreds of minor salivary glands distributed throughout the mouth.

The composition of the epithelium varies depending on the site in the oral cavity. For example, the hard palate, the gingivae, and the dorsal surface of the tongue are covered by a layer of keratinized cells, whilst the epithelium covering the soft palate, the buccal mucosa and the sublingual mucosa is non-keratinized. (Non-keratinized epithelium is more permeable to water than keratinized epithelium). Similarly, the thickness of the epithelium varies according to the site: for example, the buccal mucosa is approximately three times as thick as the sublingual mucosa (500–600 µm versus 100–200 µm) (Lee, 2001). As a result of these characteristics, the permeability of the sublingual mucosa is greater than that of the buccal mucosa, which is greater than that of the remainder of the oral mucosa (Shojaei, 1998).

The absorption of drugs across the oral mucosa involves a process of passive absorption, and may involve either the transcellular route, the paracellular route (via the intercellular spaces), or a combination of the two routes (Hao & Heng, 2003). Lipophilic drugs are predominantly absorbed using the transcellular route, whilst hydrophilic drugs are predominantly absorbed using the paracellular route. It should be noted that lipophilic drugs need to also have a degree of hydrophilicity in order to transverse the inner part of the cell (Zhang et al, 2002). Paracellular absorption is limited by the small surface area available for this type of absorption (Hao & Heng, 2003).

A number of drug factors affect the absorption of drugs across the oral mucosa, including the lipophilicity of the drug (see above), the ionized fraction of the drug (ionized drugs are less permeable), and the duration of contact with the mucosa (Hao & Heng, 2003). The amount of drug that can be absorbed is small, and so only potent drugs are suitable to be administered via the oral transmucosal route (Zhang et al, 2002).

Patients with oral mucosal disease may have altered oral transmucosal absorption (Hao & Heng, 2003). Indeed, patients may have either decreased absorption of drugs (mucosal thickening), or increased absorption of drugs (mucosal inflammation). Similarly, patients with salivary gland dysfunction may have altered oral transmucosal absorption (Hao & Heng, 2003). Thus, saliva is important in maintaining the pH of the oral cavity, which can affect the ionized fraction of the drug (Hao & Heng, 2003). Moreover, saliva may be necessary to dissolve the drug formulation (tablets, lozenges).

6.3 **Oral transmucosal administration**

The oral transmucosal route offers several advantages over the gastro-intestinal tract and other alternative routes of administration (Zhang et al, 2002):

- Acceptable to patients (non-invasive) (Walker et al, 2003)
- Convenient for patients

- Convenient for healthcare professionals
- Suitable for patients with dysphagia
- Suitable for patients with nausea and vomiting
- Suitable for patients with dysfunction of the upper gastrointestinal tract
- Potentially fast onset of action
- Avoidance of degradation by gastric acid/enzymes
- Avoidance of first pass metabolism by liver enzymes

Oral transmucosal drug delivery does not require expertise, preparation, technical equipment or supervision (of patients). Thus, oral transmucosal administration is convenient for patients, convenient for healthcare professionals, and is more cost effective than certain other (invasive) routes of administration (Zhang et al, 2002). Furthermore, oral transmucosal administration of certain drugs can provide patients with an onset of action approaching that seen with intravenous administration.

The disadvantages of the oral transmucosal route include (Zhang et al, 2002):

- Not suitable for patients with dryness of mouth
- Not suitable for patients with pathology of mouth
- Limited number suitable drugs
- Limited number suitable formulations
- Variation in oral transmucosal bioavailability

6.4 Opioids approved for oral transmucosal administration

6.4.1 Fenatyl

Fentanyl is a synthetic opioid, and an agonist at the µ receptor (analgesic effect). Fentanyl is a highly lipid-soluble, and is 80% non-ionized, making it ideally suited for transmucosal absorption.

6.4.1.1 Oral transmucosal fentanyl citrate (Actiq®)

Oral transmucosal fentanyl citrate (Actiq®) is marketed for the 'management of breakthrough pain in patients already receiving maintenance opioid therapy for chronic cancer pain' (http://www.medicines.org.uk/emc/).

Product characteristics

Oral transmucosal fentanyl citrate (OTFC) consists of a lozenge on a plastic handle (Figure 6.1). It is available in 200 µg, 400 µg, 600 µg, 800 µg, 1200 µg, and 1600 µg doses. OTFC is rubbed against the oral mucosa on the inside of the cheek, which leads to the lozenge being dissolved by saliva, and the fentanyl being absorbed through the oral mucosa.

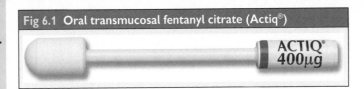

Fig 6.1 **Oral transmucosal fentanyl citrate (Actiq®)**

It usually takes ~15 min to completely dissolve the lozenge. However, patients with a dry mouth may take longer to dissolve the lozenge. The bioavailability of OTFC is ~50%: ~25% is rapidly absorbed through the oral mucosa, whilst ~25% is more slowly absorbed through the GI mucosa as a result of swallowing the drug (Mystakidou et al, 2006).

It is recommended that the lozenge be removed from the mouth if the pain gets relieved before it has completely dissolved; the remaining lozenge should not be reused, but should be dissolved under hot running water.

Clinical data

OTFC has been reported to produce meaningful pain relief after 15 min in patients with cancer pain (Coluzzi et al, 2001). The rapid onset of action is dependent on the absorption through the oral mucosa. Indeed, patients who suck the lozenge, rather than rub the lozenge against the inside of the cheek, will experience a delayed/reduced effect. The duration of analgesia is ~2 hr (Lichtor et al, 1999).

There are a number of published studies of the use of OTFC in the management of cancer-related breakthrough pain (Mystakidou et al, 2006). In general, OTFC has been found to be effective in treating breakthrough pain, and to be well tolerated by this group of patients. Moreover, the relevant Cochrane review concluded that 'OTFC is an effective treatment for breakthrough pain', and reported that OTFC produced quicker/greater analgesia than oral morphine (Figure 6.2) (Zeppetella & Ribeiro, 2006). Table 6.1 shows some data from the four randomized trials of OTFC in breakthrough cancer pain (Christie et al, 1998; Farrar et al, 1998; Portenoy et al, 1999; Coluzzi et al, 2001).

The randomized trials have demonstrated that there is no correlation between the dose of opioid needed to control the background pain and the dose of OTFC needed to control the breakthrough pain, i.e. the dose of OTFC requires individual titration (Christie et al, 1998; Portenoy et al, 1999; Coluzzi et al, 2001; Hagen et al, 2007).

The side effects of OTFC are typical of other opioid preparations, and include somnolence, nausea, vomiting and dizziness (Christie et al, 1998; Farrar et al, 1998; Portenoy et al, 1999; Coluzzi et al, 2001). Some patients are unable to use OTFC, including patients that are severely disabled (and cannot agitate the preparation), that are severely fatigued (and cannot agitate the preparation), that have ongoing oral dryness (and cannot dissolve the preparation), and

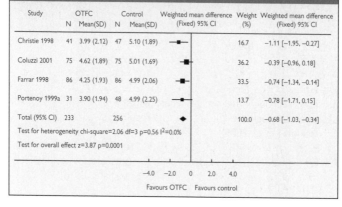

Fig 6.2 Forest plot of pain intensity difference at 15 min for oral transmucosal fentanyl citrate (reproduced with permission from Zeppetella & Ribeiro, 2006)

Study	OTFC N	Mean(SD)	Control N	Mean(SD)	Weighted mean difference (Fixed) 95% CI	Weight (%)	Weighted mean difference (Fixed) 95% CI
Christie 1998	41	3.99 (2.12)	47	5.10 (1.89)		16.7	−1.11 [−1.95, −0.27]
Coluzzi 2001	75	4.62 (1.89)	75	5.01 (1.69)		36.2	−0.39 [−0.96, 0.18]
Farrar 1998	86	4.25 (1.93)	86	4.99 (2.06)		33.5	−0.74 [−1.34, −0.14]
Portenoy 1999a	31	3.90 (1.94)	48	4.99 (2.25)		13.7	−0.78 [−1.71, 0.15]
Total (95% CI)	233		256			100.0	−0.68 [−1.03, −0.34]

Test for heterogeneity chi-square=2.06 df=3 p=0.56 I^2=0.0%

Test for overall effect z=3.87 p=0.0001

−4.0 −2.0 0 2.0 4.0

Favours OTFC   Favours control

that have ongoing oral pathology (that may affect absorption of the preparation).

6.4.1.2 Fentanyl buccal tablet (Effentora®/Fentora™)

Fentanyl buccal tablet (Effentora®/Fentora™) is marketed for the 'treatment of breakthrough pain in adults with cancer who are already receiving maintenance opioid therapy for chronic cancer pain' (http://www.medicines.org.uk/emc/). It should be noted that the product is marketed as Effentora® in Europe, and as Fentora™ in the United States of America.

Product characteristics

Fentanyl buccal tablet (FBT) is an effervescent tablet. It is available in 100 μg, 200 μg, 400 μg, 600 μg, and 800 μg doses in Europe. FBT is placed on the oral mucosa above the upper third molar (Figure 6.3), which leads to the tablet being dissolved by saliva, and the fentanyl being absorbed through the oral mucosa. FBT uses the OraVescent® Technology drug delivery system, where transient pH changes accompany an effervescent reaction resulting in both an increase in the rate of dissolution (at a lower pH) of the ionized drug, and the rate of absorption (at a higher pH) of the non-ionized drug (Figure 6.4).

It usually takes ~ 15–25 min to completely dissolve the tablet. However, patients with a dry mouth may take longer to dissolve the tablet. The bioavailability of FBT is ~ 65%: ~ 50% is rapidly absorbed through the buccal mucosa, whilst ~ 15% is more slowly absorbed through the GI mucosa as a result of swallowing the drug (Taylor, 2007).

It is recommended that the tablet is swallowed with some water if it has not completely dissolved after 30 min; the remaining tablet is likely to consist of inactive excipients rather than active fentanyl given

Table 6.1 Randomized trials of oral transmucosal fentanyl citrate

Study	Methodology	Principal outcomes
Christie et al, 1998	Multicentre, double-blind, randomized, dose titration study of OTFC. 62 cancer patients using transdermal fentanyl for background analgesia entered study.	• 76% patients titrated to an effective dose of OTFC. • No relationship was found between the successful dose of OTFC and the dose of background transdermal fentanyl. • OTFC produced significantly quicker/better analgesia than usual breakthrough analgesic. • Global satisfaction significantly higher for OTFC than usual breakthrough analgesic. • The most common adverse effects of OTFC were somnolence, nausea, dizziness and vomiting.
Portenoy et al, 1999	Multicentre, double-blind, randomized dose titration study of OTFC. 65 cancer patients using oral opioids for background analgesia entered main part of study. (67 patients were recruited to study).	• 74% patients titrated to an effective dose of OTFC. • No relationship was found between the successful dose of OTFC and the dose of background oral opioid. • OTFC produced significantly quicker/better analgesia than usual breakthrough analgesic. • Global satisfaction significantly higher for OTFC than usual breakthrough analgesic. • The most common adverse effects of OTFC were somnolence, dizziness, nausea and headache.

Farrar et al, 1998	Multicentre, double-blind, randomized, controlled, crossover trial of OTFC versus placebo. 92 cancer patients using oral opioids or transdermal fentanyl for background analgesia entered main part of study. (130 patients were recruited to study).	• OTFC produced significantly quicker / better analgesia than placebo. • Global performance of OTFC better than placebo. • Patients required significantly less additional rescue medication when using OTFC. • Most patients chose to continue with OTFC following the trial. • The most common adverse effects of OTFC were dizziness, nausea, somnolence, constipation and asthenia.
Coluzzi et al, 2001	Multicentre, double-blind, randomized, controlled, crossover trial of OTFC versus oral morphine. 93 cancer patients using oral opioids or transdermal fentanyl for background analgesia entered main part of study. (134 patients were recruited to study).	• No relationship was found between the successful dose of OTFC and the dose of background oral opioid or transdermal opioid. • OTFC produced significantly quicker / better analgesia than oral morphine. • Global performance of OTFC better than oral morphine. • Most patients chose to continue with OTFC following the trial. • The most common adverse effects of OTFC were somnolence, nausea, constipation and dizziness.

OTFC = oral transmucosal fentanyl citrate

Fig 6.3 Placement of fentanyl buccal tablet (Effentora®)

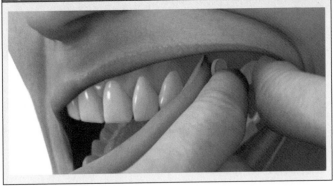

that the extent of fentanyl absorption does not appear to be affected by the time taken for tablet dissolution (Darwish *et al*, 2007).

Effentora®/Fentora™ is now approved for sublingual administration, following the demonstration that sublingual administration is essentially bioequivalent to buccal administration (Darwish *et al*, 2008).

Clinical data

FBT has been reported to produce clinically meaningful pain relief within 10 min in some patients with cancer pain (Slatkin *et al*, 2007). The rapid onset of action is dependent on the absorption through the oral mucosa.

There are a number of published studies of the use of FBT in the management of cancer-related breakthrough pain. In general, FBT has been found to be effective in treating breakthrough pain, and to be well tolerated by this group of patients. Table 6.2 shows some data from the two randomized trials of FBT in breakthrough cancer pain (Portenoy *et al*, 2006; Slatkin *et al*, 2007).

Fig 6.4 OraVescent® technology

Step 1:

$$C_6H_8O_7 \;+\; 3\,HCO_3^- \;\rightarrow\; C_6H_5O_7^- \;+\; 3\,H_2CO_3$$

Citric acid   Bicarbonate   Citrate   Carbonic acid

Production of carbonic acid reduces pH and favours dissolution of ionized fentanyl

Step 2:

$$H_2CO_3 \;\rightarrow\; H_2O \;+\; CO_2$$

Carbonic acid   Water   Carbon dioxide

Loss of CO_2 increases pH and favours absorption of non-ionized fentanyl

Table 6.2 Randomized trials of fentanyl buccal tablet

Study	Methodology	Principal outcomes
Portenoy et al, 2006	Multicentre, double-blind, randomized, controlled, crossover trial of FBT versus placebo. 77 cancer patients using oral opioids or transdermal fentanyl for background analgesia entered main part of study. (123 patients were recruited to study).	• No relationship was found between the successful dose of FBT and the dose of background oral opioid or transdermal opioid. • FBT produced significantly quicker / better analgesia than placebo. • Global performance of FBT better than placebo. • Patients required less additional rescue medication when using FBT. • The most common adverse effects of FBT were nausea, dizziness, headache, fatigue, vomiting, somnolence, constipation and asthenia.
Slatkin et al, 2007	Multicentre, double-blind, randomized, controlled, crossover trial of FBT versus placebo. 87 cancer patients using oral opioids or transdermal fentanyl for background analgesia entered main part of study. (129 patients were recruited to study).	• No relationship was found between the successful dose of FBT and the dose of background oral opioid or transdermal opioid. • FBT produced significantly quicker / better analgesia than placebo [Figure 6.6]. • Global performance of FBT better than placebo. • Patients required less additional rescue medication when using FBT. • The most common adverse effects of FBT were nausea, dizziness, fatigue, headache, vomiting and constipation.

FBT = fentanyl buccal tablet

The randomized trials have demonstrated that there is no correlation between the dose of opioid needed to control the background pain and the dose of FBT needed to control the breakthrough pain, i.e. the dose of FBT requires individual titration (Portenoy et al, 2006; Slatkin et al, 2007).

The side effects of FBT are typical of other opioid preparations, and include somnolence, nausea, vomiting and dizziness (Portenoy et al, 2006; Slatkin et al, 2007).

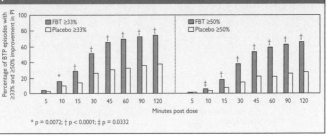

Fig 6.5 **Pain intensity differences of 33% and 50% with fentanyl buccal tablet (FBT) and placebo (reproduced with permission from Slatkin et al, 2007**

* p = 0.0072; † p < 0.0001; ‡ p = 0.0332

6.4.1.3 Sublingual fentanyl orally disintegrating tablet (Abstral®)

Sublingual fentanyl orally disintegrating tablet (Abstral®) is marketed for the 'management of breakthrough pain in adult patients using opioid therapy for chronic cancer pain' (http://www. medicines.org. uk/emc/).

Product characteristics

Sublingual fentanyl orally disintegrating tablet (ODT) is a non-effervescent tablet. It is available in 100 µg, 200 µg, 300 µg, 400 µg, 600 µg and 800 µg doses. Sublingual fentanyl ODT is placed on the oral mucosa beneath the tongue, which leads to the tablet being dissolved by saliva, and the fentanyl being absorbed through the oral mucosa. Sublingual fentanyl ODT uses a so-called 'ordered' or 'interactive' mixture to improve the absorption of the fentanyl (Bredenberg et al, 2003).

It usually takes less than a minute to completely dissolve the tablet. However, there is somewhat of a delay between the tablet dissolving in the mouth and the fentanyl reaching the circulation. The bioavailability of sublingual fentanyl ODT is thought to be ~ 70%; most is thought to be absorbed through the sublingual mucosa (Bredenberg et al, 2003).

Clinical data

Sublingual fentanyl ODT has been reported to produce clinically meaningful pain relief around 15 min in patients with cancer pain (Rauck et al, 2009). The rapid onset of action is dependent on the absorption through the oral mucosa.

Currently, there are few published studies of the use of sublingual fentanyl ODT in the management of cancer-related breakthrough pain. Table 6.3 shows some data from the one randomized trial of sublingual fentanyl ODT (Rauck et al, 2009).

Table 6.3 Randomized trials of sublingual fentanyl oral disintegrating tablet and fentanyl buccal soluble film

Study	Methodology	Principal outcomes
Rauck et al, 2009	Multicentre, double-blind, randomized, controlled, crossover trial of sublingual fentanyl ODT versus placebo. 66 cancer patients using oral opioids or transdermal fentanyl for background analgesia entered main part of study. (131 patients were recruited to study).	• Sublingual fentanyl ODT produced significantly quicker/better analgesia than placebo (Figure 6.6). • Global performance of sublingual fentanyl ODT better than placebo. • Patients required less additional rescue medication when using sublingual fentanyl ODT. • The most common adverse effects of sublingual fentanyl ODT were nausea, vomiting, somnolence, and headache.
Rauck et al, 2010	Multicentre, double-blind, randomized, controlled, crossover trial of FBSF versus placebo. 82 cancer patients using oral opioids or transdermal fentanyl for background analgesia entered main part of study. (151 patients were recruited to study).	• FBSF produced significantly quicker/better analgesia than placebo (Figure 6.7). • Global performance of FBSF better than placebo. • Patients required less additional rescue medication when using FBSF. • The most common adverse effects of FBSF were somnolence, nausea, dizziness, vomiting and headache.

ODT = oral disintegrating tablet
FBSF = fentanyl buccal soluble film

73

Fig 6.6 Pain intensity difference with sublingual fentanyl oral disintegrating tablet (ODT) and placebo (reproduced with permission from Rauck et al, 2009)

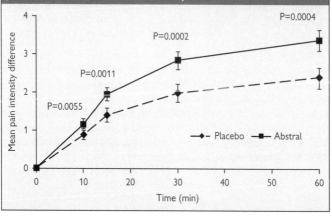

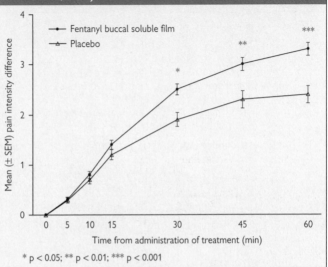

Fig 6.7 **Pain intensity difference with fentanyl buccal soluble film (FBSF) and placebo (reproduced with permission from Rauck et al, 2010)**

* p < 0.05; ** p < 0.01; *** p < 0.001

The dose of sublingual fentanyl ODT requires individual titration (in keeping with similar opioid preparations) (http://www.medicines.org.uk/emc/).

The side effects of sublingual fentanyl ODT are typical of other opioid preparations, and include nausea, vomiting, somnolence and headache (Rauck et al, 2009).

6.4.1.4 Fentanyl buccal soluble film (Breakyl®/Onsolis™)

Fentanyl buccal soluble film is indicated for the management of breakthrough pain in opioid tolerant, adult patients with cancer. It should be noted that the product will be marketed as Breakyl® in Europe, and is marketed as Onsolis™ in the United States of America. Breakyl® received regulatory approval in Europe in October 2010.

Product characteristics

Fentanyl buccal soluble film (FBSF) consists of bi-layered polymer film. It is available in 200 µg, 400 µg, 600 µg, 800 µg and 1200 µg in the United States of America. FBSF is placed on the buccal mucosa, which leads to leads to the film being dissolved by saliva, and the fentanyl being absorbed through the oral mucosa. FBSF uses the BEMA™ drug delivery system, where the outer/non drug containing layer facilitates unidirectional movement of the fentanyl from the inner/drug containing layer.

It usually takes ~ 15–30 min to completely dissolve the film. The bioavailability of FBSF is thought to be ~ 71%; most (50%) is thought to be absorbed through the sublingual mucosa (Rauck et al, 2010).

Clinical data

FBSF has been reported to produce clinically meaningful pain relief after 15 min in patients with cancer pain (Rauck et al, 2010).

Currently, there are few published studies of the use of FBSF in the management of cancer-related breakthrough pain. Table 6.3 shows some data from the one randomized trial of FBSF (Rauck et al, 2010).

The dose of FBSF requires individual titration (in keeping with similar opioid preparations).

The side effects of FBSF in are typical of other opioid preparations, and include somnolence, nausea, dizziness, vomiting, and headache (Rauck et al, 2010).

6.4.1.5 Other fentanyl products

Several authors have reported success with the sublingual adminis- tration of the parenteral preparation of fentanyl (Gardner-Nix, 2001; Zeppetella, 2001; Duncan, 2002).

6.4.2 Buprenorphine

Buprenorphine is a semi-synthetic opioid, and is a partial agonist at the μ-receptor (analgesic effect).

6.4.2.1 Sublingual buprenorphine (Temgesic®)

Sublingual buprenorphine is licensed for the 'relief of moderate to severe pain' (http://www.medicines.org.uk/emc/). It is primarily used in the management of background pain, but is also recommended for use in the management of breakthrough pain in patients receiving transdermal buprenorphine (Anonymous, 2005).

Product characteristics

Sublingual buprenorphine is available in 200 μg and 400 μg doses. Sublingual buprenorphine is placed under the tongue, which allows the tablet to dissolve in the pool of saliva in the floor of the mouth, and the buprenorphine to be absorbed through the mucosa of the floor of the mouth.

Pharmacokinetic profile

Buprenorphine is highly lipophilic, and is well absorbed across mucosal membranes. The percentage absorption is ~ 55% after sub- lingual administration (Figure 6.8) (Weinberg et al, 1988), although it is somewhat less after buccal administration (Davis, 2005). However, the rate of systemic absorption can be slow: peak plasma concentrations occur 0.5–3 hr after sublingual administration (Davis, 2005).

Clinical data

The reported onset of action of sublingual buprenorphine is ~15–30 min, the peak analgesic effect is at ~60–120 min, and the duration of action is ~8 hr (Thompson, 1990). (The delayed peak analgesic effect, and the long duration of action, is disadvantageous for the treatment of breakthrough pain).

There have been numerous studies of the use of sublingual buprenorphine in the management of cancer-related pain (Davis, 2005). The majority of these studies report its use for background pain, but some studies also report its use for breakthrough pain (with the transdermal buprenorphine patch) (Sittl *et al*, 2003; Sorge & Sittl, 2004). However, there appear to have been no studies of the specific use of sublingual buprenorphine in the management of cancer-related breakthrough pain.

The adverse effects encountered with buprenorphine are typical of those encountered with opioid analgesics. Buprenorphine is reported to cause more dizziness, nausea and vomiting than morphine (Davis, 2005). However, it is reported to cause less respiratory depression and constipation than morphine (Davis, 2005). It should be noted that the effects of buprenorphine are only partially reversed by opioid antagonists (e.g. naloxone) (Anonymous, 2005).

6.5 **Other opioids for transmucosal administration**

A variety of other opioids have been subject to oral transmucosal administration. However, many of these opioids are not very lipophilic and, therefore, not suited for buccal or sublingual administration. Figure 6.8 shows the percentage absorption for selected opioids administered by the sublingual route (Weinberg *et al*, 1988).

6.5.1 **Morphine**

Morphine is not very lipophilic, and 90% of its molecules are ionized at the normal oral pH (Coluzzi, 1998). Thus, the physicochemical properties of morphine are not favourable for oral transmucosal absorption. Indeed, only 18% of the dose is absorbed after sublingual administration (Figure 6.8) (Weinberg *et al*, 1988).

A review of the literature concluded that 'the limited clinical data do not provide compelling evidence for the effectiveness of sublingual morphine for the rapid relief of pain in cancer patients' (Coluzzi, 1998). Moreover, morphine's long duration of action (~ 4hr) makes it less than ideal as a rescue medication for breakthrough pain.

6.5.2 **Diamorphine**

Diamorphine is a semi-synthetic analogue of morphine, and is much more lipophilic than morphine. Indeed, ~ 30% of the dose is absorbed after sublingual administration (Figure 6.8) (Weinberg *et al*, 1988).

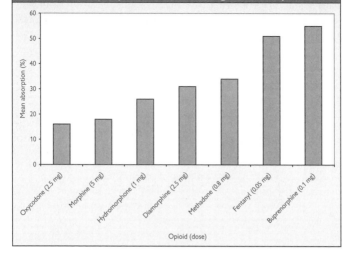

Fig 6.8 Absorption of opioid analgesics after sublingual administration (adapted from Weinberg et al, 1988)

It appears that there is no published data on the use of oral transmucosal diamorphine in the management of breakthrough pain. However, buccal diamorphine has been used in the management of breakthrough pain in paediatric palliative care (Finella Craig, personal communication). Nevertheless, diamorphine's long duration of action (~ 4hr) makes it less than ideal as a rescue medication for breakthrough pain.

6.5.3 Hydromorphone
Hydromorphone has a relatively low lipid solubility, which results in limited transmucosal absorption (Figure 6.8) (Weinberg et al, 1988). The low bioavailability and long duration of action of hydromorphone (~ 4hr) mean that this drug is also not suited for the treatment of breakthrough pain.

6.5.4 Oxycodone
Oxycodone has a very low lipid solubility, which results in very limited transmucosal absorption (Figure 6.8) (Weinberg et al, 1988). Again, the low bioavailability, and long duration of action of oxycodone (~ 4hr) mean that this drug is not suited for the treatment of breakthrough pain.

6.5.5 Methadone
Methadone is a lipophilic drug, which is well absorbed across mucosal membranes. The percentage absorption is 35% after sublingual administration (Figure 6.8) (Weinberg et al, 1988). Indeed, the sublingual bioavailability is reported to be similar to the oral bioavailability (McQuay et al, 1986).

Sublingual methadone has been reported to be effective in the management of cancer-related breakthrough pain (Hagen *et al*, 2007; Hagen *et al*, 2010). Interestingly, some patients reported an analgesic effect within 5 min of use of sublingual methadone. However, the use of sublingual methadone is likely to be limited by the pharmacokinetics of methadone per se (i.e. long $t_{\frac{1}{2}}$).

6.5.6 **Alfentanil**

Alfentanil is a synthetic opioid analgesic, which is chemically similar to fentanyl. It is less lipophilic than fentanyl, but has a more rapid onset of action, and shorter duration of action when given parenterally (Scholz *et al*, 1996). For example, when given intravenously, the onset of action is < 2 min, and the duration of action is 10 min (Twycross *et al*, 2002). These characteristics suggest that alfentanil could be particularly helpful in the management of breakthrough pain.

A parenteral preparation of alfentanil has been reported to be effective and well tolerated when administered bucally/sublingually in a small case series of patients with cancer-related breakthrough pain (Duncan, 2002). Interestingly, patients preferred buccal administration of the preparation. It should be noted, that the main reason for choosing alfentanil in this series was the availability of a suitable (concentrated) preparation of alfentanil, i.e. only small volumes of alfentanil were required to be administered.

6.5.7 **Sufentanil (not available in the UK)**

Sufentanil is another synthetic opioid analgesic, which is chemically similar to fentanyl. It is more lipophilic than fentanyl, and has a more rapid onset of action, and shorter duration of action when given parenterally (Scholz *et al*, 1996). Again, these characteristics suggest that sufentanil could be particularly helpful in the management of breakthrough pain.

There have been a number of published reports supporting the role of sublingual sufentanil in the management of breakthrough pain (Kunz *et al*, 1993; Gardner-Nix, 2001). In the study by Gardner Nix, the onset of action was reported to be between 4–6 min, and the duration of action 35 min (Gardner-Nix, 2001). Indeed, some patients required a combination of the short acting sufentanil, and a longer acting oral opioid (morphine, hydromorphone), to control some longer lasting episodes of breakthrough pain. Again, the main reason for choosing sufentanil in this series was the availability of a suitable (concentrated) preparation of sufentanil.

References

Anonymous (2005) *British National Formulary 50*. BMJ Publishing Group Ltd and Royal Pharmaceutical Society of Great Britain, London.

Bredenberg, S., Duberg, M., Lennernas, B. *et al* (2003) In vitro and in vivo evaluation of a new sublingual tablet system for rapid oromucosal absorption using fentanyl citrate as the active substance. *European Journal of Pharmaceutical Sciences*, **20**, 327–34.

Christie, J.M., Simmonds, M., Patt, R. *et al* (1998) Dose-titration, multicenter study of oral transmucosal fentanyl citrate for the treatment of breakthrough pain in cancer patients using transdermal fentanyl for persistent pain. *Journal of Clinical Oncology*, **16**, 3238–45.

Coluzzi, P.H. (1998) Sublingual morphine: efficacy reviewed. *Journal of Pain and Symptom Management*, **16**, 184–92.

Coluzzi, P.H., Schwartzberg, L., Conroy, Jr J.D. *et al* (2001) Breakthrough cancer pain: a randomized trial comparing oral transmucosal fentanyl citrate (OTFC) and morphine sulfate immediate release (MSIR). *Pain*, **91**, 123–30.

Darwish, M., Kirby, M., Jiang, J.G. (2007) Effect of buccal dwell time on the pharmacokinetic profile of fentanyl buccal tablet. *Expert Opinion in Pharmacotherapy*, **8**, 2011–6.

Darwish, M., Kirby, M., Jiang, J.G., Tracewell, W., Robertson, Jr P. (2008) Bioequivalence following buccal and sublingual placement of fentanyl buccal tablet 400 µg in healthy subjects. *Clinical Drug Investigation*, **28**, 1–7.

Davis, M.P. (2005) Buprenorphine in cancer pain. *Supportive Care in Cancer*, **13**, 878–87.

Duncan, A. (2002) The use of fentanyl and alfentanil sprays for episodic pain. *Palliative Medicine*, **16**, 550.

Farrar, J.T., Cleary, J., Rauck, R., Busch, M., Nordbrock, E. (1998) Oral transmucosal fentanyl citrate: randomized, double-blinded, placebo-controlled trial for treatment of breakthrough pain in cancer patients. *Journal of the National Cancer Institute*, **90**, 611–6.

Gardner-Nix J (2001) Oral transmucosal fentanyl and sufentanil for incident pain. *Journal of Pain and Symptom Management*, **22**, 627–30.

Hagen, N.A., Fisher, K., Victorino, C., Farrar, J.T. (2007) A titration strategy is needed to manage breakthrough cancer pain effectively: observations from data pooled from three clinical trials. *Journal of Palliative Medicine*, **10**, 47–55.

Hagen, N.A., Fisher, K., Stiles, C. (2007) Sublingual methadone for the management of cancer-related breakthrough pain: a pilot study. *Journal of Palliative Medicine*, **10**, 331–7.

Hagen, N.A., Moulin, D.E., Brasher, P.M. *et al* (2010) A formal feasibility study of sublingual methadone for breakthrough cancer pain. *Palliative Medicine*, **24**, 696–706.

Hao, J., Heng, P.W. (2003) Buccal delivery systems. *Drug Development and Industrial Pharmacy*, **29**, 821–32.

Kunz, K.M., Theisen, J.A., Schroeder, M.E. (1993) Severe episodic pain: management with sublingual sufentanil. *Journal of Pain and Symptom Management*, **8**, 189.

Lee, V.H. (2001) Mucosal drug delivery. *Journal of the National Cancer Institute, Monographs*, (29), 41–4.

Lichtor, J.L., Sevarino, F.B., Joshi, G.P., Busch, M.A., Nordbrock, E., Ginsberg, B. (1999) The relative potency of oral transmucosal fentanyl citrate compared with intravenous morphine in the treatment of moderate to severe postoperative pain. *Anesthesia and Analgesia*, **89**, 732–8.

McQuay, H.J., Moore, R.A., Bullingham, R.E. (1986) Sublingual morphine, heroin, methadone and buprenorphine: kinetics and effects. In Foley, K.M., Inturrisi, C.E., ed. *Opioid Analgesics in the Management of Clinical Pain. Advances in Pain Research and Therapy.* Volume 8, pp. 407–12. Raven Press, New York.

Mystakidou, K., Katsouda, E., Parpa, E., Vlahos, L., Tsiatas, M.L. (2006) Oral transmucosal fentanyl citrate: overview of pharmacological and clinical characteristics. *Drug Delivery*, **13**, 269–76.

Portenoy, R.K., Payne, R., Coluzzi, P. *et al* (1999) Oral transmucosal fentanyl citrate (OTFC) for the treatment of breakthrough pain in cancer patients: a controlled dose titration study. *Pain*, **79**, 303–12.

Portenoy, R.K., Taylor, D., Messina, J., Tremmel, L. (2006) A randomized, placebo-controlled study of fentanyl buccal tablet for breakthrough pain in opioid-treated patients with cancer. *Clinical Journal of Pain*, **22**, 805–11.

Rauck, R.L., Tark, M., Reyes, E. *et al* (2009) Efficacy and long-term tolerability of sublingual fentanyl orally disintegrating tablet in the treatment of breakthrough cancer pain. *Current Medical Research and Opinion*, **25**, 2877–85.

Rauck, R., North, J., Gever, L.N., Tagarro, I., Finn, A.L. (2010) Fentanyl buccal soluble film (FBSF) for breakthrough pain in patients with cancer: a randomized, double-blind, placebo-controlled study. *Annals of Oncology*, **21**, 1308–14.

Scholz, J., Steinfath, M., Schulz, M. (1996) Clinical pharmacokinetics of alfentanil, fentanyl and sufentanil. An Update. *Clinical Pharmacokinetics*, **31**, 275–92.

Shojaei, A.H. (1998) Buccal mucosa as a route for systemic drug delivery: a review. *Journal of Pharmacy and Pharmaceutical Sciences*, **1**, 15–30.

Sittl, R., Griessinger, N., Likar, R. (2003) Analgesic efficacy and tolerability of transdermal buprenorphine in patients with inadequately controlled chronic pain related to cancer and other disorders: a multicenter, randomized, double-blind, placebo-controlled trial. *Clinical Therapeutics*, **25**, 150–68.

Slatkin, N.E., Xie, F., Messina, J., Segal, T.J. (2007) Fentanyl buccal tablet for relief of breakthrough pain in opioid-tolerant patients with cancer-related chronic pain. *Journal of Supportive Oncology*, **5**, 327–34.

Sorge, J., Sittl, R. (2004) Transdermal buprenorphine in the treatment of chronic pain: results of a phase III, multicenter, randomized, double-blind, placebo-controlled study. *Clinical Therapeutics*, **26**, 1808–20.

Taylor, D.R. (2007) Fentanyl buccal tablet: rapid relief from breakthrough pain. *Expert Opinion on Pharmacotherapeutics*, **8**, 3043–51.

Thompson, J.W. (1990) Clinical pharmacology of opioid agonists and partial agonists. In Doyle, D., ed. *Opioids in the Treatment of Cancer Pain*. pp. 17–38. Royal Society of Medicine Services Ltd, London.

Twycross, R., Wilcock, A., Charlesworth, S., Dickman, A. (2002) *Palliative Care Formulary*, 2nd edn. Radcliffe Medical Press, Abingdon.

Walker, G., Wilcock, A., Manderson, C., Weller, R., Crosby, V. (2003) The acceptability of different routes of administration of analgesia for breakthrough pain. *Palliative Medicine*, **17**, 219–21.

Weinberg, D.S., Inturrisi, C.E., Reidenberg, B. *et al* (1988) Sublingual absorption of selected opioid analgesics. *Clinical Pharmacology and Therapeutics*, **44**, 335–42.

Zeppetella, G. (2001) Sublingual fentanyl citrate for cancer-related breakthrough pain: a pilot study. *Palliative Medicine*, **15**, 323–8.

Zeppetella, G., Ribeiro, M.D. (2006) Opioids for the management of breakthrough (episodic) pain in cancer patients. *Cochrane Database of Systematic Reviews*, (**1**), CD004311.

Zhang, H., Zhang, J., Streisand, J.B. (2002) Oral mucosal drug delivery: clinical pharmacokinetics and therapeutic applications. *Clinical Pharmacokinetics*, **41**, 661–80.

Chapter 7

Intranasal and intrapulmonary opioids

Key points

- The suitability of different opioid delivery routes depends on a number of physicochemical and pharmaceutical factors
- The intranasal route can be associated with rapid onset of analgesia, and intranasal fentanyl-based formulations are commercially available
- The intrapulmonary route also has the potential for rapid onset of analgesia. Clinical studies are ongoing of fentanyl-based formulations.

7.1 Introduction

Opioids can be administered via a number of different routes in the management of breakthrough pain. The decision to use a particular route depends on variety of factors, including the availability of a suitable opioid formulation, the appropriateness of the route (and the inappropriateness of other routes), and the acceptability of the route. This chapter will discuss the role of the intranasal, the intrapulmonary and the transdermal routes of administration.

7.2 Intranasal opioids

The nose has a relatively small surface area for absorption ($\sim$ 150–180 cm^2). However, the nasal epithelium is highly permeable, and also highly perfused with blood. The latter factors help to facilitate the absorption of drugs. A special feature of the nose is its close connection to the brain in the olfactory area (i.e. absence of the normal blood – brain barrier); this may enable a fraction of the drug to directly enter the intrathecal space (Dale et al, 2002a).

The nose can only accommodate volumes of 150–200 µl in each nostril, which restricts the opioid formulations suitable for intranasal administration. In addition, there is a continuous turnover/flow of mucus within the nose, which limits the time available for the drug to be absorbed to ~ 15 min. Intranasal administration negates the phenomenon of hepatic first pass metabolism.

The intranasal route is simple, does not necessarily require any specialized equipment, and can be used by both patients and their non-professional caregivers. Thus, opioids can be delivered by traditional spray bottles, and also by syringes fitted with atomizers. The intranasal route may be inappropriate in some patients with local disease of the nose, and may be difficult to use in patients that are uncooperative.

The intranasal route is a reasonably acceptable route of administration for the treatment of breakthrough pain. For example, Walker et al reported that 50% of patients thought that the route was acceptable for pain that was mild to moderate in nature, whilst 68% thought that the route was acceptable for pain that was severe in nature (Walker et al, 2003). A number of different reasons were given for not wanting to use the intranasal route (see Tables 4.3 and 4.4) (Walker et al, 2003).

7.2.1 Fentanyl

7.2.1.1 Intranasal fentanyl citrate (Instanyl®)

Intranasal fentanyl citrate (Instanyl®) is marketed for the 'management of breakthrough pain in adults already receiving maintenance opioid therapy for chronic cancer pain' (http://www.medicines.org. uk/emc/).

Product characteristics

Instanyl® consists of a simple solution of fentanyl citrate, and comes in a standard 100 µl/spray dispenser. It is available in 50 µg/spray, 100 µg/spray, and 200 µg/spray doses. Instanyl® is delivered into the nasal passages with the patient in an upright position (see Figure 7.2), and the fentanyl is absorbed into the systemic circulation through the nasal mucosa. The bioavailability of this product is reported to be 89% (Foster et al, 2008).

Clinical data

Instanyl® has been reported to produce clinically meaningful pain within 10 min (Kress et al, 2009; Mercadante et al, 2009), with some patients reporting a response at 5 min post dosage (Figure 7.2) (Mercadante et al, 2009). The duration of analgesia is ~ 1 hr in the post operative setting (Christrup et al, 2008).

Table 7.1 gives an overview of the data from randomized controlled trials involving the use of Instanyl® for cancer-related breakthrough pain (Kress et al, 2009; Mercadante et al, 2009). In general the product has been found to be very effective, and more effective than both placebo (Kress et al, 2009) and oral transmucosal fentanyl

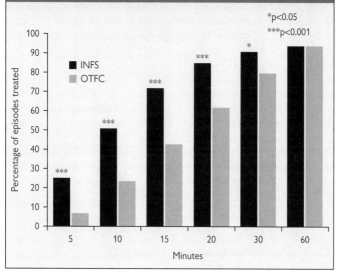

Fig 7.1 Time to 33% reduction in pain intensity with intranasal fentanyl spray (INFS) and oral transmucosal fentanyl citrate (OTFC) (reproduced with permission from Mercadante et al, 2009)

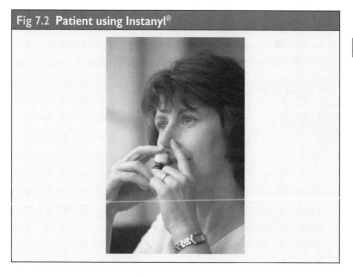

Fig 7.2 Patient using Instanyl®

Table 7.1 Randomized controlled trials of Instanyl®

Study	Methodology	Principal outcomes
Kress et al, 2009	Multicentre, double-blind, randomized, controlled, crossover trial of Instanyl® versus placebo. 113 cancer patients using oral opioids or transdermal fentanyl for background analgesia were randomized. (120 patients were enrolled into study).	• Instanyl® produced significantly quicker/better analgesia than placebo. • Patients required somewhat less additional rescue medication when using Instanyl®. • The most common adverse effects of Instanyl® were nausea, constipation and asthenia. • Majority of patients continued into the extension study
Mercadante et al, 2009	Multicentre, open-label, randomized, controlled, crossover trial of Instanyl® versus OTFC. 139 cancer patients using oral opioids or transdermal fentanyl for background analgesia were randomized. (196 patients were enrolled into study).	• Instanyl® produced significantly quicker/better analgesia than OTFC. • Patients required slightly more additional rescue medication when using Instanyl®. • Majority of patients preferred Instanyl®. • The most common adverse effects of Instanyl® were nausea, vomiting and constipation.

OTFC = oral transmucosal fentanyl citrate

citrate (Mercadante et al, 2009). Moreover, the product was well tolerated, and caused typical opioid-related side effects with minimal local toxicity. Of note, Instanyl® appears to be suitable for use in patients with both the common cold and allergic rhinitis (Nave et al, 2009a; Nave et al, 2009b).

7.2.1.2 Fentanyl Pectin Nasal Spray (PecFent®)

Fentanyl pectin nasal spray (PecFent®) is marketed for the 'management of breakthrough pain (BTP) in adults already receiving maintenance opioid therapy for chronic cancer pain' (http://www.medicines.org.uk/emc/).

Product characterisitics

PecFent® consists of a solution of fentanyl citrate and a proprietary pectin-based transmucosal delivery system (PecSys®), and comes in a bespoke 100 µl/spray dispenser. It is available in 100 µg/spray, and 400 µg/spray doses. PecFent® is delivered into the nasal passages with the patient in an upright position, and the fentanyl is absorbed into the systemic circulation through the nasal mucosa.

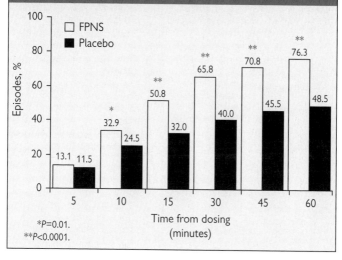

Fig 7.3 Percentage of episodes with ≥ 2 point reduction in pain intensity with fentanyl pectin nasal spray (FPNS) and placebo (reproduced with permission from Portenoy et al, 2010)

*P=0.01.
**P<0.0001.

Clinical data

PecFent® has been reported to produce clinically meaningful pain within 10 min (Figure 7.3) (Portenoy et al, 2010; Davies et al, 2011).

Table 7.2 gives an overview of the data from randomized controlled trials involving the use of PecFent® for cancer-related breakthrough pain (Portenoy et al, 2010; Davies et al, 2011). In general the product has been found to be very effective, and more effective than both placebo (Portenoy et al, 2010) and oral morphine sulphate (Davies et al, 2011). Moreover, the product was well tolerated, and caused typical opioid-related side effects with minimal local toxicity. Of note, PecFent® appears to be suitable for use in patients with allergic rhinitis, although the concomitant use of oxymetazoline does influence the pharmacokinetics, i.e. decreased Cmax, increased Cmax (http://www.medicines.org.uk/emc/).

7.2.1.3 Other fentanyl products

Several authors have reported success with the intranasal administration of non-commercial formulations of fentanyl (Zeppetella, 2000a; Zeppetella, 2000b; Duncan, 2002), as well as alfentanil (Duncan, 2002), and sufentanil (not available in the UK) (Jackson et al, 2002; Good et al, 2009).

7.2.2 Morphine

Several authors have reported success with the intranasal administration of non-commercial formulations of morphine (Pavis et al,

Table 7.2 Randomized controlled trials of PecFent®

Study	Methodology	Principal outcomes
Portenoy et al, 2010	Multicentre, double-blind, randomized, controlled, crossover trial of PecFent® versus placebo. 83 cancer patients using oral opioids or transdermal fentanyl for background analgesia were randomized. (139 patients were enrolled into study).	• PecFent® produced significantly quicker/better analgesia than placebo. • Patients required significantly less additional rescue medication when using PecFent®. • The most common adverse effects of Instanyl® were nausea, vomiting and dizziness. • Majority of patients continued into the extension study
Davies et al, 2011	Multicentre, open-label, randomized, controlled, crossover trial of PecFent® versus oral morphine sulphate. 84 cancer patients using oral opioids or transdermal fentanyl for background analgesia were randomized. (135 patients were enrolled into study).	• PecFent® produced significantly quicker/better analgesia than oral morphine sulphate. • (The most common adverse effects of PecFent® were nausea, vomiting, somnolence and constipation).

2002; Fitzgibbon et al, 2003), and diamorphine (Kendall et al, 2003). However, the long duration of effect of these opioids is a significant disadvantage.

7.2.3 Methadone

Methadone has been found to be too much of an irritant for intra-nasal administration (Dale et al, 2002b).

7.3 Intrapulmonary opioids

The lungs have an extremely large surface area for absorption. Moreover, the alveolar surface is highly permeable, and also highly perfused with blood. (The lungs are the most highly perfused organs in the body). All of these factors help to facilitate the absorption of drugs.

The intrapulmonary route is simple, does not necessarily require specialized equipment, and can be used by both patients and their non-professional caregivers. Thus, opioids can be delivered by traditional nebulizers, and other inhalation devices (e.g. metered dose inhalers, dry powder inhalers). The intrapulmonary route may be inappropriate in some patients with local disease of the lung, and may be difficult to use in patients that are uncooperative.

The intrapulmonary route is a reasonably acceptable route of administration for the treatment of breakthrough pain. For example, Walker *et al* reported that 60% of patients thought that the route was acceptable for pain that was mild to moderate in nature, whilst 75% thought that the route was acceptable for pain that was severe in nature (Walker *et al*, 2003). A number of different reasons were given for not wanting to use the intrapulmonary route (see Tables 4.3 and 4.4) (Walker *et al*, 2003).

7.3.1 **Fentanyl**

Zeppetella reported on a small, case series of intrapulmonary fentanyl for cancer-related breakthrough pain (Zeppetella, 2000a). The first patient was treated with 25 µg fentanyl, achieved good pain control within 15 min, and did not develop any local or systemic adverse effects. The second patient was treated with 125 µg fentanyl, achieved good pain control within 15 min, and again did not develop any local or systemic adverse effects.

It should be noted that a number of pharmaceutical companies are currently developing intrapulmonary, fentanyl-based formulations for the management of breakthrough cancer pain.

7.4 **Transdermal opioids**

At present, transdermal administration has no role to play in the treatment of breakthrough pain. However, new patch technology (iontophoretic technology) may alter the current state of affairs (Sinatra, 2005).

References

Christrup, L.L., Foster, D., Popper, L.D., Troen, T., Upton, R. (2008) Pharmacokinetics, efficacy, and tolerability of fentanyl following intranasal versus intravenous administration in adults undergoing third-molar extraction: a randomized, double-blind, double-dummy, two-way, crossover study. *Clinical Therapeutics*, **30**, 469–81.

Dale, O., Hjortkjaer, R., Kharasch, E.D. (2002a) Nasal administration of opioids for pain management in adults. *Acta Anaesthesiologica Scandinavica*, **46**, 759–70.

Dale, O., Hoffer, C., Sheffels, P., Kharasch, E.D. (2002b) Disposition of nasal, intravenous, and oral methadone in healthy volunteers. *Clinical Pharmacology and Therapeutics*, **72**, 536–45.

Davies, A., Sitte, T., Elsner, F., Reale, C., Espinosa, J., Brooks, D. *et al* (2011) Consistency of efficacy, patient acceptability, and nasal tolerability of fentanyl pectin nasal spray compared with immediate-release morphine sulfate in breakthrough cancer pain. *Journal of Pain and Symptom Management*, **41**, 358–66.

Duncan, A. (2002) The use of fentanyl and alfentanil sprays for episodic pain. *Palliative Medicine*, **16**, 550.

Fitzgibbon, D., Morgan, D., Dockter, D., Barry, C., Kharasch, E.D. (2003) Initial pharmacokinetic, safety and efficacy evaluation of nasal morphine gluconate for breakthrough pain in cancer patients. *Pain*, **106**, 309–15.

Foster, D., Upton, R., Christrup, L., Popper, L. (2008) Pharmacokinetics and pharmacodynamics of intranasal versus intravenous fentanyl in patients with pain after oral surgery. *Annals of Pharmacotherapy*, **42**, 1380–7.

Good, P., Jackson, K., Brumley, D., Ashby, M. (2009) Intranasal sufentanil for cancer-associated breakthrough pain. *Palliative Medicine*, **23**, 54–8.

Jackson, K., Ashby, M., Keech, J. (2002) Pilot dose finding study of intranasal sufentanil for breakthrough and incident cancer-associated pain. *Journal of Pain and Symptom Managment*, **23**, 450–2.

Kendall, C.E., Davies, A.N., Forbes, K. (2003) Nasal diamorphine for 'breakthrough pain' in palliative care – a promising approach to a difficult problem [Abstract 509]. In *Proceedings of 8th Congress of the European Association for Palliative Care*. p. 92. 2–5th April, Hague, Netherlands.

Kress, H.G., Oronska, A., Kaczmarek, Z., Kaasa, S., Colberg, T., Nolte, T. (2009) Efficacy and tolerability of intranasal fentanyl spray 50 to 200 microg for breakthrough pain in patients with cancer: a phase III, multinational, randomized, double-blind, placebo-controlled, crossover trial with a 10-month, open-label extension treatment period. *Clinical Therapeutics*, **31**, 1177–91.

Mercadante, S., Radbruch, L., Davies, A., Poulain, P., Sitte, T., Perkins, P. et al (2009) A comparison of intranasal fentanyl spray with oral transmucosal fentanyl citrate for the treatment of breakthrough cancer pain: an open-label, randomised, crossover trial. *Current Medical Research and Opinion*, **25**, 2805–15.

Nave, R., Sides, E.H., Colberg, T., Meng, X., Lahu, G., Schmitt, H. (2009a) Pharmacokinetics of intranasal fentanyl spray (INFS) in subjects with common cold. *European Journal of Pain*, **13**(Suppl 1), S207.

Nave, R., Sides, E.H., Colberg, T., Meng, X., Lahu, G., Schmitt, H. (2009b) Pharmacokinetics of intranasal fentanyl spray (INFS) in subjects with seasonal allergic rhinitis with and without prior administration of oxymetazoline. *European Journal of Pain*, 13(Suppl 1), S207.

Pavis, H., Wilcock, A., Edgecombe, J. et al (2002) Pilot study of nasal morphine-chitosan for the relief of breakthrough pain in patients with cancer. *Journal of Pain and Symptom*, **24**, 598–602.

Portenoy, R.K., Burton, A.W., Gabrail, N., Taylor, D. (2010) A multicenter, placebo-controlled, double-blind, multiple-crossover study of fentanyl pectin nasal spray (FPNS) in the treatment of breakthrough cancer pain. *Pain*, **151**, 617–24.

Sinatra, R. (2005) The fentanyl HCl patient-controlled transdermal system (PCTS): an alternative to intravenous patient-controlled analgesia in the postoperative setting. *Clinical Pharmacokinetics*, **44**(Suppl 1), 1–6.

Walker, G., Wilcock, A., Manderson, C., Weller, R., Crosby, V. (2003) The acceptability of different routes of administration of analgesia for breakthrough pain. *Palliative Medicine*, **17**, 219–21.

Zeppetella, G. (2000a) Nebulized and intranasal fentanyl in the management of cancer-related breakthrough pain. *Palliative Medicine*, **14**, 57–8.

Zeppetella, G. (2000b) An assessment of the safety, efficacy, and acceptability of intranasal fentanyl citrate in the management of cancer-related breakthrough pain: a pilot study. *Journal of Pain and Symptom Management*, **20**, 253–8.

Chapter 8

Non-opioid analgesics

Key points

- Breakthrough pains have diverse characteristics as they span all pain phenomena, and can effectively involve every class of drug used in analgesia
- Non-opioid drugs can be used to treat opioid poorly-responsive pain or to supplement opioid use
- Both analgesics and drugs whose primary function is not analgesia may be used
- Paracetamol, non-steroidal anti-inflammatory drugs, midazolam, ketamine, and NO are all potential treatments of breakthrough pain.

8.1 Introduction

Non opioid analgesics have an established role in the management of background pain (WHO, 1996), and have an important role in the management of breakthrough pain. Non opioid analgesics may be taken on a regular basis ('around the clock' medication) and/or may be taken on an as required basis ('rescue' medication). Chapter 4 discusses the use of non-opioids as around the clock medication, whilst this chapter discusses the use of specific non opioids as rescue medication.

Recently, Davies *et al* reported on the strategies used by 320 European oncology patients to manage their breakthrough pain episodes (Davies *et al*, 2011). All patients were using opioid analgesics as rescue medication, whilst 90 (28%) patients were also using non-opioid analgesics as rescue medication. A variety of different non opioid analgesics were being used (Table 8.1), and some patients were using more than one type of non-opioid analgesic. However, the most common medication was paracetamol (acetaminophen).

Table 8.1 Non-opioids used by patients to manage break-through pain episodes (Davies *et al*, 2011)	
Non-opioid analgesic*	**Number of patients (n = 320)**
None	230 (72.0%)
Paracetamol	57 (18.0%)
Systemic non-steroidal anti-inflammatory drug (NSAID)	21 (6.5%)
Topical non-steroidal anti-inflammatory drug (NSAID)	8 (2.5%)
Benzodiazepine	8 (2.5%)
Antispasmodic (smooth muscle relaxant)	5 (1.5%)
Anticonvulsant	2 (0.5%)
Antipsychotic	1 (0.5%)
Local anaesthetic	1 (0.5%)
Oxygen	1 (0.5%)
* Patient could be using more than one medication	

8.2 **Paracetamol (acetaminophen)**

Paracetamol is licensed for the treatment of mild to moderate pain (Anonymous, 2005). Its analgesic action appears to be related to inhibition of prostaglandin production in the central nervous system (rather than in the periphery) (Twycross *et al*, 2002).

Paracetamol is generally used as around the clock medication, although it may be also be used as rescue medication. Paracetamol is recommended in the World Health Organization pain guidelines (WHO, 1996); it can be used in isolation at step 1, or in combination with opioids at step 2/3, of the World Health Organization analgesic ladder.

The evidence for the use of paracetamol in the management of cancer pain is somewhat limited (McNichol *et al*, 2005). Stockler *et al* reported an additive effect when paracetamol was added to a regimen containing opioids for moderate to severe pain (Stockler *et al*, 2004). However, Axelsson and Borup Christensen reported no effect when paracetamol was removed from a regimen containing opioids for moderate to severe pain (Axelsson & Borup Christensen, 2003).

Data from acute pain studies suggests a number needed to treat (NNT) of 3.8 for a single dose of 1000 mg paracetamol (Moore *et al*, 2003). The NNT for paracetamol is greater than the NNTs for the non-steroidal anti-inflammatory drugs. Moreover, Ventafridda *et al* reported that cancer patients found paracetamol less effective than non-steroidal anti-inflammatory drugs in a study of step 1 of the World Health Organization analgesic ladder (Ventafridda *et al*, 1990).

Paracetamol can be given via the oral, rectal and intravenous routes of administration (Anonymous, 2005). The onset of action of oral paracetamol is 15–30 min, and the duration of action is 4–6 hr (Twycross *et al*, 2002). There are no contra-indications to the use of paracetamol. Side effects are uncommon: reported side effects include rashes, thrombocytopenia, and leucopenia. Serious liver damage may follow an overdose of paracetamol, although it may be prevented by administration of acetylcysteine (Anonymous, 2005).

8.3 **Non-steroidal anti-inflammatory drugs (NSAIDs)**

NSAIDs are licensed for the treatment of variety of painful conditions, including inflammatory conditions (e.g. rheumatoid arthritis), degenerative conditions (e.g. osteoarthritis), other painful conditions (e.g. dysmenorrhoea), and post-operative pain (Anonymous, 2005). Their analgesic action appears to be related to inhibition of prostaglandin production both at the site of injury/disease (reducing inflammation), and also in the central nervous system (reducing central sensitization) (Twycross *et al*, 2002).

NSAIDs inhibit prostaglandin production by inhibiting the enzyme cyclo-oxygenase (COX). COX is present in a number of different forms (Dickman & Ellershaw, 2004). Conventional NSAIDs inhibit both COX-1 and COX-2, whilst the newer 'coxibs' specifically inhibit COX-2. It was thought that COX-2 was an inducible (by inflammation) enzyme, and that inhibition of COX-2 would be associated with minimal systemic adverse events. However, it is now known that COX-2 is also a constitutive enzyme, and that inhibition of COX-2 is associated with significant systemic adverse events (see below).

NSAIDs are generally used as around the clock medication, although they may be also be used as rescue medication. NSAIDs are recommended in the World Health Organization pain guidelines (WHO, 1996); they can be used in isolation at step 1, or in combination with opioids at step 2/3, of the World Health Organization analgesic ladder. Indeed, NSAIDs have an established role as an opioid-sparing manoeuvre (Mercadante & Portenoy, 2001).

Systematic reviews of oral NSAIDs have confirmed benefits in cancer pain (Eisenberg *et al*, 1994; McNichol *et al*, 2005). In the original systematic review, NSAIDs were found to be more effective than placebo, and there appeared to be no benefit to the combination of a NSAID and an opioid for mild to moderate pain (Eisenberg et al, 1994). In the subsequent systematic review, NSAIDs were again found to be more effective than placebo, and there appeared to be a slight benefit to the combination of a NSAID and an opioid (McNichol et al, 2005). However, the authors of this review were unable to comment on the relative efficacy of individual NSAIDs (i.e. calculate NNTs), or the relative tolerability of individual NSAIDs (i.e. calculate numbers needed to harm/NNHs) (McNicol et al, 2005).

Data from acute pain studies suggests NNTs of 2–3 for a single dose of the common oral NSAIDs (e.g. diclofenac, ibuprofen) (Moore et al, 2003). It should be noted that the NNTs for NSAIDs are lower than the NNTs for other analgesic drugs (e.g. opioids for mild to moderate pain). Data from other studies suggests a combined NNT of 3.1 for topical NSAIDs (Moore et al, 1998).

NSAIDs can be given via the oral, oral transmucosal, rectal, intravenous, intramuscular, subcutaneous, and transdermal routes of administration (Anonymous, 2005; Twycross et al, 2002). The onset of action, and duration of action, of certain oral NSAIDs is shown in Table 8.2. There are a number of contra-indications to the use of NSAIDs, including hypersensitivity to aspirin/NSAIDs, coagulation defects, active peptic ulcer disease (all NSAIDs), previous

Table 8.2 Clinical features of specific non steroidal anti-inflammatory drugs (Micromedex® database; Twycross et al, 2002)

Non steroidal anti-inflammatory drug	Onset of action (oral route)	Duration of action (oral route)	Comments
Ibuprofen	15–25 min	4–6 hr	Peak effect: 30–90 min
Diclofenac	30 min	8 hr	
Ketorolac	30 min	6 hr	Peak effect: 3 hr Onset of action for iv/im route: 30 min
Naproxen	30–60 min	6–8 hr	Duration of action for repeated doses: > 12 hr
Meloxicam	90 min	(24 hr)	Onset of action for im route: 80 min
Celecoxib	45–60 min	(24 hr)	

peptic ulcer disease (conventional NSAIDs), ischaemic heart disease (coxibs), cerebrovascular disease (coxibs), peripheral arterial disease (coxibs), and moderate to severe congestive cardiac failure (coxibs) (Anonymous, 2005). In addition, there are a number of relative contra-indications, relating to the known adverse effects of NSAIDs (see below) (Anonymous, 2005).

Side effects are relatively common. The major side effects of conventional NSAIDs are hypersensitivity reactions (e.g. bronchospasm), gastrointestinal problems (e.g. peptic ulceration), renal problems (e.g. renal failure), and cardiovascular problems (e.g. congestive cardiac failure) (Anonymous, 2005). Gastrointestinal problems are a major cause of morbidity/mortality. However, gastrointestinal problems may be reduced by prescribing lower risk NSAIDs (e.g. ibuprofen), by co-prescribing appropriate gastroprotection (e.g. proton pump inhibitors), and addressing other risk factors (Dickman & Ellershaw, 2004). The major side effects of coxibs are cardiovascular problems (e.g. ischaemic heart disease) (Anonymous, 2005), although coxibs can also cause gastrointestinal problems (e.g. peptic ulceration) (Anonymous, 2005). It should be noted that NSAIDs may cause a variety of other (less serious) side effects (Anonymous, 2005).

8.4 Other non-opioids

8.4.1 Midazolam

Midazolam is a parenteral benzodiazepine, which is licensed for sedation, pre-medication for anaesthesia, and induction of anaesthesia (Anonymous, 2005). Its mechanism of action involves binding to the $GABA_A$ receptor, thereby enhancing the inhibitory effect of GABA (Twycross et al, 2002).

As discussed, midazolam is licensed for sedation. It is used to sedate patients prior to investigative procedures (e.g. endoscopy) (Dundee et al, 1984), and also prior to therapeutic procedures (e.g. wound dressing) (Jacox et al, 1994). Apart from its use in procedural pain, there is little evidence to support a wider role in the management of breakthrough pain. However, there has been a report of its use in the treatment of refractory incident pain secondary to bone metastases (del Rosario et al, 2001), and there is the potential for its use in the management of breakthrough pain secondary to muscle spasm (Twycross et al, 2002).

Midazolam is only available as a parenteral preparation in the United Kingdom. Nevertheless, the parenteral preparation may be administered via enteral routes (i.e. buccal, rectal). It has a short onset of action (intravenous - 2-3 min; subcutaneous – 5–10 min), but a relatively long duration of action (~ 4 hr) (Twycross et al, 2002).

Contra-indications to the use of midazolam include acute pulmonary insufficiency, and severe respiratory depression (Anonymous, 2005). The side effects of midazolam include confusion, ataxia, amnesia, headache, euphoria, hallucinations, fatigue, dizziness, vertigo, involuntary movements, paradoxical excitement, aggression, dysarthria, respiratory depression, and cardiorespiratory arrest (Anonymous, 2005). In addition, there is the potential to develop tolerance, and dependence, to the drug; these problems only occur during chronic administration of the drug.

8.4.2 **Ketamine**

Ketamine is a parenteral anaesthetic agent, which is licensed for induction and maintenance of anaesthesia (Anonymous, 2005), but which is also used for treatment of difficult-to-control pain (Twycross et al, 2002). The analgesic effect of ketamine is thought to be related to blockade of the N-methyl D-aspartame receptor (and reduction of central sensitization/'wind-up'), although it may be related to a number of other actions including an effect on descending inhibitory pathways (Meller, 1996).

Ketamine is employed in anaesthetic doses in the management of procedural pain (Jacox et al, 1994). Carr et al reported a small double-blind, randomized, controlled, crossover trial of intranasal ketamine in the management of predominantly non-malignant breakthrough pain (Carr et al, 2004). The intranasal ketamine was found to be generally very effective (and more effective than placebo); the onset of pain relief was within 10 min, the peak effect occurred at 40 min, and the duration of pain relief was at least 60 min. The intranasal ketamine was also found to be generally well tolerated; side effects included fatigue, dizziness, feeling of unreality, and change in taste.

Ketamine has been given by the oral, intramuscular (licensed), intravenous (licensed), subcutaneous, intranasal, and spinal routes of administration. The side effects of ketamine include involuntary muscle contractions, hypertension (previous history is a relative contra-indication), tachycardia, and hallucinations (previous history is a relative contraindication) (Anonymous, 2005). Hallucinations can be prevented/treated with benzodiazepines (e.g. diazepam) (Anonymous, 2005).

8.4.3 **Nitrous oxide**

Nitrous oxide is an inhalational anaesthetic, which is licensed for maintenance of anaesthesia, and management of pain (sub-anaesthetic doses) (Anonymous, 2005). Its mechanism of action has not been completely elucidated: one hypothesis is that nitrous oxide causes the release of opioid peptides in the periaqueductal grey area of the midbrain, which leads to activation of descending noradrenergic pathways, which in turn leads to modulation of pain impulses in the dorsal horn of the spinal cord (Entonox® Reference Guide).

As discussed, nitrous oxide is licensed for the management of pain. It is used to treat patients with pain related to pathological processes (e.g. trauma) (Donen *et al*, 1982), and also pain due to therapeutic procedures (e.g. wound dressings) (Jacox *et al*, 1994). Apart from its use in procedural pain, there is some evidence to support a wider role in the management of breakthrough pain. Thus, there is a small case series (Keating & Kundrat, 1996), and a small double-blind, randomised, controlled, crossover trial (Parlow *et al*, 2005), which support the use of nitrous oxide in the management of breakthrough pain. However, there is another small case series, which does not support the use of nitrous oxide in the management of breakthrough pain (Enting *et al*, 2002).

Nitrous oxide is co-administered with oxygen (50:50 mixture for analgesia): it comes in a portable gas cylinder with a breath-activated valve, and may be used with either a face mask or a mouth piece. It has a short onset of action (<< 1 min), a quick time to peak effect (2 min), and a short duration of action (5-40 min: subjective measures-objective measures) (Entonox® Reference Guide).

Contra-indications to the use of nitrous oxide include the presence of a pneumothorax: the nitrous oxide can diffuse into the pneumothorax, causing an increase in the volume/pressure of the pneumothorax (Anonymous, 2005). The side effects of nitrous oxide include sedation (7.6%), dizziness (10.3%), nausea (5.7%), excitation (3.7%) and 'numbness' (0.3%) (Entonox® Reference Guide). Nitrous oxide can interfere with vitamin B12, and chronic usage may result in megaloblastic anaemia, and neurological problems (polyneuropathy, spinal cord degeneration) (Anonymous, 2005; Doran *et al*, 2004). In addition, there is the potential to develop tolerance to the drug; this problem may occur during acute administration of the drug (Ramsay *et al*, 2005).

8.4.4 **Other agents**

It should be noted that a variety of other sedative and anaesthetic agents have also been used to treat procedural pain (e.g. propofol, barbiturates) (Jacox *et al*, 1994).

References

Anonymous (2005) *British National Formulary 50*. BMJ Publishing Group Ltd and Royal Pharmaceutical Society of Great Britain, London.

Axellson, B., Borup, Christensen S. (2003) Is there an additive analgesic effect of paracetamol at step 3? A double-blind randomized controlled study. *Palliative Medicine*, **17**, 724–5.

Carr, D.B., Goudas, L.C., Denman, W.T. *et al* (2004) Safety and efficacy of intranasal ketamine for the treatment of breakthrough pain in patients with chronic pain: a randomized, double-blind, placebo-controlled, cross-over study. *Pain*, **108**, 17–27.

Davies, A., Zeppetella, G., Andersen, S. *et al* (2011) Multi-centre European study of breakthrough cancer pain: pain characteristics and patient perceptions of current and potential management strategies. *European Journal of Pain*, **15**, 756–63.

del Rosario, M.A., Martin, A.S., Ortega, J.J., Feria, M. (2001) Temporary sedation with midazolam for control of severe incident pain. *Journal of Pain and Symptom Management*, **21**, 439–42.

Dickman, A., Ellershaw, J. (2004) NSAIDs: gastroprotection or selective COX-2 inhibitor? *Palliative Medicine*, **18**, 275–86.

Donen, N., Tweed, W.A., White, D., Guttormson, B., Enns, J. (1982) Prehospital analgesia with Entonox. *Canadian Anaesthetists' Society Journal*, **29**, 275–9.

Doran, M., Rassam, S.S., Jones, L.M., Underhill, S. (2004) Toxicity after inhalation of nitrous oxide for analgesia. *British Medical Journal*, **328**, 1364–5.

Dundee, J.W., Halliday, N.J., Harper, K.W., Brogden, R.N. (1984) Midazolam. A review of its pharmacological properties and therapeutic use. *Drugs*, **28**, 519–43.

Eisenberg, E., Berkey, C.S., Carr, D.B., Mosteller, F., Chalmers, T.C. (1994) Efficacy and safety of nonsteroidal antiinflammatory drugs for cancer pain: a meta-analysis. *Journal of Clinical Oncology*, **12**, 2756–65.

Enting, R.H., Oldenmenger, W.H., van der Rijt, C.C., Koper, P., Lieverse, J., Sillevis, S.P. (2002) Nitrous oxide is not beneficial for breakthrough cancer pain. *Palliative Medicine*, **16**, 257–9.

Jacox, A., Carr, D.B., Payne, R. *et al* (1994) *Management of Cancer Pain*. Agency for Health Care Policy and Research, Rockville.

Keating, H.J., Kundrat, M. (1996) Patient-controlled analgesia with nitrous oxide in cancer pain. *Journal of Pain and Symptom Management*, **11**, 126–30.

McNicol, E., Strassels, S.A., Goudas, L., Lau, J., Carr, D.B. (2005) NSAIDS or paracetamol, alone or combined with opioids, for cancer pain. *Cochrane Database of Systematic Reviews*, (2), CD005180.

Meller, S.T. (1996) Ketamine: relief from chronic pain through actions at the NMDA receptor? *Pain*, **68**, 435–6.

Mercadante, S., Portenoy, R.K. (2001) Opioid poorly-responsive cancer pain. Part 3. Clinical strategies to improve opioid responsiveness. *Journal of Pain and Symptom Management*, **21**, 338–54.

Moore, R.A., Tranmer, M.R., Carroll, D., Wiffen, P.J., McQuay, H.J. (1998) Quantitative systematic review of topically applied non-steroidal antiinflammatory drugs. *British Medical Journal*, **316**, 333–8.

Moore, A., Edwards, J., Barden, J., McQuay, H. (2003) *Bandolier's Little Book of Pain*. Oxford University Press, Oxford.

Parlow, J.L., Milne, B., Tod, D.A., Stewart, G.I., Griffiths, J.M., Dudgeon, D.J. (2005) Self-administered nitrous oxide for the management of incident pain in terminally ill patients: a blinded case series. *Palliative Medicine*, **19**, 3–8.

Ramsay, D.S., Leroux, B.G., Rothen, M., Prall, C.W., Fiset, L.O., Woods, S.C. (2005) Nitrous oxide analgesia in humans: acute and chronic tolerance. *Pain*, **114**, 19–28.

Stockler, M., Vardy, J., Pillai, A., Warr, D. (2004) Acetaminophen (paracetamol) improves pain and well-being in people with advanced cancer already receiving a strong opioid regimen: a randomized, double-blind, placebo-controlled, cross-over trial. *Journal of Clinical Oncology*, **22**, 3389–94.

Twycross, R., Wilcock, A., Charlesworth, S., Dickman, A. (2002) *Palliative Care Formulary*, 2nd edn. Radcliffe Medical Press, Abingdon.

Ventafridda, V., De Conno, F., Panerai, A.E., Maresca, V., Monza, G.C., Ripamonti, C. (1990) Non-steroidal anti-inflammatory drugs as the first step in cancer pain therapy: double-blind, within patient study comparing nine drugs. *Journal of International Medical Research*, **18**, 21–9.

World Health Organization (1996) *Cancer Pain Relief*, 2nd edn. World Health Organization, Geneva.

Chapter 9

Other therapeutic interventions

Key points

- A wide variety of non-pharmacological interventions have been used to treat cancer-related pain
- Patients often use non-pharmacological interventions in conjunction with pharmacological interventions
- Anaesthetic interventions can be used to treat difficult pain problems associated with breakthrough pain episodes
- Anaesthetic interventions are usually intended to be an adjuvant to systemic analgesic treatment.

9.1 Introduction

A variety of non-pharmacological interventions have been reported to be useful in treating breakthrough pain, although most of them have not been subjected to rigorous scientific investigation:

- Rubbing/massage (Fine & Busch, 1998; Swanwick et al, 2001)
- Application of heat (Fine & Busch, 1998; Swanwick et al, 2001)
- Application of cold (Fine & Busch, 1998; Petzke et al, 1999)
- Distraction techniques (Petzke et al, 1999; Portenoy, 1997)
- Relaxation techniques (Fine & Busch, 1998; Portenoy, 1997)
- Hypnotherapy/hypnosis (Wild & Espie, 2004)
- Transcutaneous electrical nerve stimulation (TENS) (Figure 9.1) (Zeppetella, 2010) – see below
- Acupuncture (Zeppetella, 2010) – see below.

In a recent study, 88% of patients had identified an intervention that at least 'sometimes' improved their breakthrough pain: in 34% of these patients the treatment was a non-pharmacological intervention, and in another 18% of these patients the treatment was a combination of a pharmacological and a non-pharmacological intervention (Davies et al, 2011). A variety of different non-pharmacological

Table 9.1 Non-pharmacological interventions used by patients to manage breakthrough pain episodes (Davies et al, 2011)

Intervention*	Number of patients (n = 320)
None	159 (49.5%)
Change of position	28 (8.5%)
Physical support	7 (2.0%)
Rest/sleep	41 (13.0%)
Movement/exercise	16 (5.0%)
Heat	72 (22.5%)
Cold	3 (1.0%)
Rubbing/massage	11 (3.5%)
Transcutaneous electrical nerve stimulation (TENS)	12 (3.5%)
Relaxation/visualization	10 (3.0%)
Distraction	8 (2.5%)
Miscellaneous other interventions	8 (2.5%)
*Patient could be using more than one intervention	

Fig 9.1 Physio-Med TPN 200 PP TENS machine

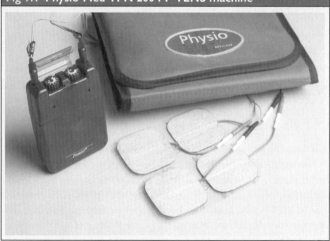

interventions were utilised, and in some cases more than one non-pharmacological intervention was utilized at some time (Table 9.1) (Davies *et al*, 2011).

As discussed above, there is little scientific evidence to support the utilization of these interventions. However, there is enough anecdotal evidence to support at least a trial of these interventions, particularly as these interventions are generally well tolerated by patients (and generally acceptable/available to patients). Non-pharmacological interventions may be used in isolation, or in combination with pharmacological interventions. In the latter scenario, the non-pharmacological interventions may produce an analgesic effect in advance of the pharmacological interventions.

9.1.1 Transcutaneous electrical nerve stimulation (TENS)

There is limited scientific evidence to support the use of TENS in the management of cancer pain (Bercovitch & Cherny, 2010). Nevertheless, TENS is often used as an adjuvant treatment for background cancer pain, and sometimes used as an adjuvant treatment for breakthrough cancer pain. Thus, Davies *et al* reported that 3.5% of the northern European patients with breakthrough cancer pain in their study used TENS to manage their breakthrough pain episodes (Davies *et al*, 2011).

9.1.2 Acupuncture

Similarly, there is limited scientific evidence to support the use of acupuncture in the management of cancer pain (Filshie & Thompson, 2010). Nevertheless, acupuncture is often used as an adjuvant treatment for background cancer pain, and has been suggested as an adjuvant treatment for breakthrough cancer pain (Zeppetella, 2010). However, Davies *et al* found that none of the northern European patients with breakthrough cancer pain in their study used acupuncture to manage their breakthrough pain episodes (Davies *et al*, 2011; Andrew Davies, personal communication).

9.2 Anaesthetic strategies

Anaesthetic interventions are usually utilized as an adjuvant to pharmacological treatment. Thus, these interventions are generally indicated in patients with pain that is poorly responsive to systemic analgesics, and/or in patients with intolerable side effects from systemic analgesics (Swarm *et al*, 2010). Currently, these interventions have a somewhat limited role in the management of cancer pain. For example, only 11% patients required anaesthetic interventions to help to control their pain in a validation study of the World Health Organization analgesic guidelines (Zech *et al*, 1995).

The decision to utilize an anaesthetic intervention depends on a number of factors: 1) pain-related factors – is the pain amenable to an anaesthetic intervention?; 2) patient-related factors – is the patient suitable for the proposed intervention/is the patients willing to undertake the proposed intervention?; 3) healthcare professional-related factors – is the anaesthetist adequately trained/experienced to undertake the intervention?; 4) health service-related factors – is the supporting team adequately trained/experienced to manage the aftercare for the intervention?; 5) the cost of the anaesthetic intervention; and 6) the availability/suitability of alternative interventions.

Anaesthetic interventions are usually utilized in patients with uncontrolled background pain, but they are sometimes used in patients with uncontrolled breakthrough pain. A variety of different techniques are available (Swarm *et al*, 2010):

- Peripheral (local anaesthetic) nerve blockade – see below
- Neuraxial analgesia delivery – see below
- Neuromodulation (e.g. TENS, spinal cord stimulation)
- Neuroablation – neuroablation (neurolytic blockade) involves the physical interruption or destruction of the neurones involved in conducting painful impulses

  1. Neurolytic blockade of peripheral nerves
  2. Neurolytic blockade of sympathetic nervous system (e.g. celiac plexus block, lumbar sympathetic block)
  3. Neurolytic blockade of central nervous system (e.g. cervical cordotomy, intrathecal neurolysis).

9.2.1 **Peripheral (local anaesthetic) nerve blockade**

Peripheral (local anaesthetic) nerve blockade is usually used to manage uncontrolled background pain, although it is sometimes used to manage breakthrough pain. Techniques include bolus injections of local anaesthetic (with or without corticosteroid), and continuous infusions of local anaesthetic via an indwelling catheter.

In terms of breakthrough pain, Mercadante *et al* have reported on the successful use of a continuous infusion of local anaesthetic to block the suprascapular nerve in a patient with volitional incident pain (movement-related pain) from a bone metastasis within the scapula (Mercadante *et al*, 1995).

9.2.2 **Neuraxial analgesia delivery**

Again, neuraxial analgesia delivery is usually used to manage uncontrolled background pain, although it is sometimes used to manage breakthrough pain. Techniques include continuous infusions of various analgesics (opioid analgesics, local anaesthetic, other agents) via an indwelling catheter in the epidural space ('epidural'), or the subarachnoid space ('intrathecal').

In terms of breakthrough pain, Kalso et al reported a decrease in volitional incident pain (movement-related pain) on switching patients from oral administration of opioids to epidural administration of opioids (Kalso et al, 1996). Additionally, Mercadante et al have reported on the successful use of intrathecal boluses of local anaesthetic to treat breakthrough pain in patients receiving intrathecal infusions of local anaesthetic and opioids for their background pain (Mercadante et al, 2005a; Mercadante et al, 2005b).

9.3 **Other interventional strategies**

Movement-related (volitional incident) pain, secondary to metastatic bone disease, is a common phenomenon. Moreover, studies suggest that this can be the most difficult type of breakthrough pain to manage (Hwang et al, 2003). A variety of interventional techniques have been reported to be useful in treating pain secondary to metastatic bone disease, although most of these interventional techniques have not been subjected to rigorous scientific investigation:

- Non-surgical stabilization (Figure 4.2) (Mercadante et al, 2002)
- Surgical stabilization (Figure 4.1b) (Mercadante & Arcuri, 1998)
- Corticosteroid instillation (Rousseff & Simeonov, 2004)
- Alcohol instillation (Gangi et al, 1996)
- Phenol instillation (Gangi et al, 1996)
- Cryoablation (Callstrom et al, 2006)
- Radiofrequency ablation (Goetz et al, 2004)
- Laser ablation (Callstrom et al, 2006)
- Cementoplasty/vertebroplasty (Gangi et al, 2003) – this technique involves injecting methylmethacrylate cement into the affected bone
- Balloon kyphoplasty (Fourney et al, 2003) – this technique is similar to vertebroplasty, but involves initially inflating a balloon within the affected bone (to improve the alignment of the bone, and also to create a cavity for the cement within the bone).
- MR-guided focused ultrasound surgery (Liberman et al, 2008).

It should be noted that many of these patients may also benefit from strategies to minimize the amount of movement required, such as provision of simple adaptations to their surroundings and provision of additional practical support with the activities of daily living (Mercadante & Arcuri 1998).

References

Bercovitch, M., Cherny, N.I. (2010) Treating pain with transcutaneous electrical nerve stimulation. In Hanks, G., Cherny, N.I., Christakis, N.A., Fallon, M., Kaasa, S., Portenoy, R.K., ed. *Oxford Textbook of Palliative Medicine*, 4th edn, pp. 763–8. Oxford University Press, Oxford.

Callstrom, M.R., Charboneau, J.W., Goetz, M.P. *et al* (2006) Image-guided ablation of painful metastatic bone tumors: a new and effective approach to a difficult problem. *Skeletal Radiology*, **35**, 1–15.

Davies, A., Zeppetella, G., Andersen, S. *et al* (2011) Multi-centre European study of breakthrough cancer pain: pain characteristics and patient perceptions of current and potential management strategies. *European Journal of Pain*, **15**, 756–63.

Filshie, J., Thompson, J.W. (2010) Acupuncture. In Hanks, G., Cherny, N.I., Christakis, N.A., Fallon, M., Kaasa, S., Portenoy, R.K., ed. *Oxford Textbook of Palliative Medicine*, 4th edn, pp. 768–84. Oxford University Press, Oxford.

Fine, P.G., Busch, M.A. (1998) Characterization of breakthrough pain by hospice patients and their caregivers. *Journal of Pain and Symptom Management*, **16**, 179–83.

Fourney, D.R., Schomer, D.F., Nader, R. *et al* (2003) Percutaneous vertebroplasty and kyphoplasty for painful vertebral body fractures in cancer patients. *Journal of Neurosurgery*, **98**(1 Suppl), 21–30.

Gangi, A., Dietemann, J.L., Schultz, A., Mortazavi, R., Jeung, M.Y., Roy, C. (1996) Interventional radiologic procedures with CT guidance in cancer pain management. *Radiographics*, **16**, 1289–1304.

Gangi, A., Guth, S., Imbert, J.P., Marin, H., Dietemann, J.L. (2003) Percutaneous vertebroplasty: indications, technique, and results. *Radiographics*, **23**, e10.

Goetz, M.P., Callstrom, M.R., Charboneau, J.W. *et al* (2004) Percutaneous image-guided radiofrequency ablation of painful metastases involving bone: a multicenter study. *Journal of Clinical Oncology*, **22**, 300–6.

Hwang, S.S., Chang, V.T., Kasimis, B. (2003) Cancer breakthrough pain characteristics and responses to treatment at a VA medical center. *Pain*, **101**, 55–64.

Kalso, E., Heiskanen, T., Rantio, M., Rosenberg, P.H., Vainio, A. (1996) Epidural and subcutaneous morphine in the management of cancer pain: a double-blind cross-over study. *Pain*, **67**, 443–9.

Liberman, B., Gianfelice, D., Inbar, Y. *et al* (2008) Pain palliation in patients with bone metastases using MR-guided focused ultrasound surgery: a multicenter study. *Annals of Surgical Oncology*, **16**, 140–6.

Mercadante, S., Sapio, M., Villari, P. (1995) Suprascapular nerve block by catheter for breakthrough shoulder cancer pain. *Regional Anesthesia*, **20**, 343–6.

Mercadante, S., Arcuri, E. (1998) Breakthrough pain in cancer patients: pathophysiology and treatment. *Cancer Treatment Reviews*, **24**, 425–32.

Mercadante, S., Radbruch, L., Caraceni, A. *et al* (2002) Episodic (breakthrough) pain. Consensus Conference of an Expert Working Group of the European Association for Palliative Care. *Cancer*, **94**, 832–9.

Mercadante, S., Ferrera, P., Villari, P., Arcuri, E. (2005a) Local anaesthetics for breakthrough pain in patients receiving intrathecal treatment fot cancer pain management. *Anesthesia and Analgesia*, **100**, 1540.

Mercadante, S., Arcuri, E., Ferrera, P., Villari, P., Mangione, S. (2005b) Alternative treatments of breakthrough pain in patients receiving spinal analgesics for cancer pain. *Journal of Pain and Symptom Management*, **30**, 485–91.

Petzke, F., Radbruch, L., Zech, D., Loick, G., Grond, S. (1999) Temporal presentation of chronic cancer pain: transitory pains on admission to a multidisciplinary pain clinic. *Journal of Pain and Symptom Management*, **17**, 391–401.

Portenoy, R.K. (1997) Treatment of temporal variations in chronic cancer pain. *Seminars in Oncology*, **5**, S16–7-12.

Rousseff, R.T., Simeonov, S. (2004) Intralesional treatment in painful rib metastases. *Palliative Medicine*, **18**, 259.

Swanwick, M., Haworth, M., Lennard, R.F. (2001) The prevalence of episodic pain in cancer: a survey of hospice patients on admission. *Palliative Medicine*, **15**, 9–18.

Swarm, R.A., Karanikolas, M., Cousins, M.J. (2004) Injections, neural blockade, and implant therapies for pain control. In Hanks, G., Cherny, N.I., Christakis, N.A., Fallon, M., Kaasa, S., Portenoy, R.K., ed. *Oxford Textbook of Palliative Medicine*, 4th edn, pp. 734–55. Oxford University Press, Oxford.

Wild, M.R., Espie, C.A. (2004) The efficacy of hypnosis in the reduction of procedural pain and distress in pediatric oncology: a systematic review. *Journal of Developmental and Behavioral Pediatrics*, **25**, 207–13.

Zech, D.F., Grond, S., Lynch, J., Hertel, D., Lehmann, K.A. (1995) Validation of World Health Organization Guidelines for cancer pain relief: a 10-year prospective study. *Pain*, **63**, 65–76.

Zeppetella, G. (2010) Breakthrough pain. In Hanks, G., Cherny, N.I., Christakis, N.A., Fallon, M., Kaasa, S., Portenoy, R.K., ed. *Oxford Textbook of Palliative Medicine*, 4th edn, pp. 654–61. Oxford University Press, Oxford.

Index

111